What Every Woman Must Know

On The Inside Press

Ojai, CA

To my wife, Kate,

who is my love and friend.

A perfect example of womanhood.

What Every Woman Must Know

DR. VLADIMIR GORDIN

Published by **On The Inside Press**

.

Author: Dr. Vladimir Gordin
Phone: (847) 243-2110
Email: *info@gordinmedical.com*
Websites:
www.GordinMedical.com
www.HealMeVladimir.com
www.Health1240.com

Book Design:
Writers for the Future, LLC.
Email: *Writers.for.the.Future@gmail.com*
Web: FutureWrit.com, AlexanderPhoenix.com

A complete listing of picture credits can be found at the back of this book.

ISBN 978-0-9882652-0-2

Table Of Contents

Chapter 1:

An Introduction to Alternative Therapy

Why is conventional medicine a failure and how can alternative medicine help save lives?

Americans almost exclusively use Modern Medicine for treatment, and the US government endorses this practice without thinking twice. The concept of alternative therapy and alternative medicine were often laughed at until recently, but practitioners and researchers of modern medicine have started to appreciate the various advantages of alternative therapy.

One reason for alternative therapy not getting the respect it deserves is the relative lack of research based proof for the efficacy of alternative medicine. Often, this has lead to advocates of modern medicine to ignore or dismiss it. Alternative therapy has been around for several thousands of years, long before many ancient civilizations were setting up roots. Those were the days when humans were hunters and, despite a certain primitive lifestyle, managed to amass impeccable knowledge about the medicinal powers of certain plant and animal byproducts.

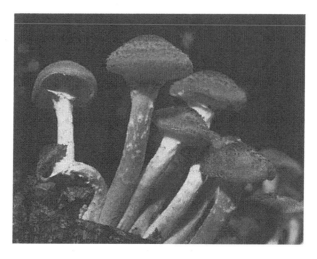

How Old Is Alternative Medicine?

Most of us realize that alternative medicine was a prominent treatment method for many ancient cultures and its history is several thousands of years old. However, it is hard to believe that the oldest traces of alternative medicine date back to 60,000 years. This is long before many ancient civilizations were even born!

A good example is a Neanderthal tomb excavated in 1963, which is estimated to be at least 60,000 years old. This tomb contained many herbs that are believed to be offerings for the deceased. Shanidar IV, the Neanderthal tomb in Iraq, contained herbs such as Centaurea solstitialis, Senecio-type, Ephedra altissima, Achillea-type, Muscari-type and Althea-type.

Centaurea solstitialis is also known as the yellow star thistle, and has been used historically in the treatment of ulcers. Senecio is no more than the common daisy, and it is not only a diuretic and a diaphoretic, but can also be used in the treatment of female diseases. Ephedra altissima, also sometimes called the sea-grape, is an interesting herb used since ancient times in the treatment of respiratory disorders, like asthma and hay fever. It can also be used to treat the common cold. Achillea, more commonly called the yarrow, has been used since ancient times as a diaphoretic agent. It also has a stimulating and astringent effect. Muscari is also known as the Grape Hyacinthm, and can be used as an antioxidant and as a rich source of Vitamin C. It can also be used in poultice for irritated skin. Althea is commonly known as the marshmallow plant, and the juice thereof can be used to treat ulcers of the mouth and throat, as well as ulcers of the gastric system.

The medicinal effects of these plants were researched later and it was found that they have significant therapeutic effects. It is probably these medicinal effects that led Neanderthals to keep them in a tomb.[1]

It is clear that alternative therapy's powers were discerned by humans several thousands of years ago. Powerful treatment systems, comparable to modern medicine, were therefore developed in many countries. A good example is Ayurveda, the traditional Indian treatment method with herbs and animal properties. Ayurveda is still practiced extensively in India and it is interesting to note that its usage is widespread in the South Indian state of Kerala that has living standards comparable to West.[2]

---

[1] NCBI. Accessed May 15, 2012.
http://www.ncbi.nlm.nih.gov/pubmed/1548898
[2] JStor. Accessed May 15, 2012.
http://www.jstor.org/discover/10.2307/4372130?uid=3738256&uid=2&uid=4&sid=47698967570967

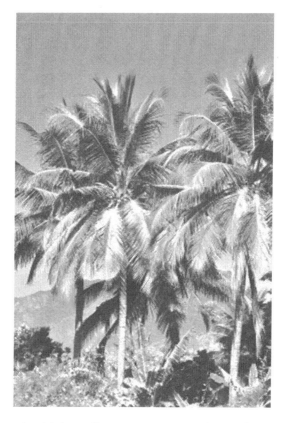

Kerala has the highest literacy rate in India and it is the only Indian state where the male to female ratio is high (1000 males to 1054 females). The state has a very long life expectancy, low mortality rates and a sub-replacement fertility rate lower than the United States. Although it a well-educated state with extensive access to modern medicine and hospitals, Keralites embraces Ayurveda and uses it for the treatment of many ailments.

Dr. Vladimir Gordin

Why Does Modern Medicine Need Alternatives?

The contributions of modern medicine are appreciable in many areas of diagnosis and treatment, particularly emergency care. However, diseases presenting as part of emergency medicine account for merely 20% of the disorders in the United States. For the majority of diseases (at least 80%), at least one form of alternative therapy is proven to be an effective treatment. Compared to modern medicine, alternative medicine, particularly chiropractic medicine, has almost no side effects. This fact gives alternative treatment methods an extra edge.

Even worse, modern medicine is not always effective in completely eliminating an illness without some side effects. It recurrently fails to comprehend the fact that a series of disorders we encounter are a result of our diet, habits and living conditions. One of the first people to shed some light on this was Dr. Weston A Price, who was ignored by Western medicine. With research, he proved that a good number of chronic disorders in Western society are a result of our diet and these disorders can't be found in 26 primitive societies. [3]

The Drug Problem in Modern Medicine

It doesn't take a rocket scientist to observe that modern medicine is advancing every day. Nevertheless, it seems that things are not as charming as we perceive and modern medicine is in crisis. This is a matter of concern for most of us: the so-called 'drug problem' refers to the significant lack of medicinal drugs to treat illness.

---

[3] Natural health information. Accessed May 15, 2012.
http://www.natural-health-information-centre.com/modern-medicine.html

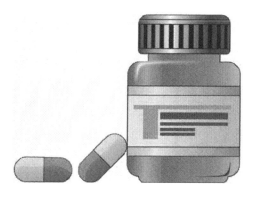

The drug problem is much complex than you think, and has several factors contributing to it. The research and development pipeline in modern medicine is very long. Several certifications have to be obtained from concerned authorities and multiple tests and studies have to be carried out. Without these expensive steps, a new drug will never see the light. This process easily lasts for several years, and extends to decades in some cases!

In simple terms, finding a new drug to treat an illness and releasing it to the masses is not as easy as one might think, and it is a process that lasts for many years. With the World Health Organization's awareness campaigns and involvement, even developing countries have many stringent regulations regarding new drugs and the path they have to take before winding up in a pharmacy. The end result of these regulations is a drug crisis.

Additionally, drug resistance is a very unfortunate downside of modern medicine, and this has not been helped by the phenomenon of medicinal abuse. Constant abuse of antibiotics causes drug resistance and many developing countries are often blamed for not taking any action against hospitals that promote the over usage of such antibiotics. Still, the startling fact is that even developed countries like United States are a victim of drug resistance. [4]

Drug resistance can shoot your health in the dark because it is pretty common for some microorganisms to develop resistance. Basically, these organisms become resistant to drugs that are already harmful to our body and taking these drugs in increased doses will only worsen the situation.

Sleeping sickness, once a widespread disease, is not very common today but the drug resistance of a parasite called *Trypanosoma brucei* is very alarming. Drugs used in the treatment of sleeping sickness (pentamidine, eflornithine, melasoprol, nifurtimox and suramin) are not only expensive but they are highly toxic too.

To cure sleeping disorder, a patient needs to undergo prolonged treatment. The increased dosages of the toxic drugs used for treatment can seriously damage a person's health.[5]

Herbs Are More Powerful Than One Might Think

Traditional medicine was viewed with skepticism by Western society mostly because many treatments originated in places that are today's developing nations. These countries have not advanced in many areas of science and technology, and

---

[4] SciDev. Accessed May 15, 2012.
http://www.scidev.net/en/health/antibiotic-resistance/opinions/biomed-analysis-end-complacency-on-drug-resistance-1.html
[5] SciDev. Accessed May 15, 2012.
http://www.scidev.net/en/health/antibiotic-resistance/news/sleeping-sickness-drug-resistance-mechanism-identified.html

Western society has a tendency to overlook their treatment methods as a result.

A good example is Chinese Sweet Wormwood, from which the medicine for malaria, Artemisinin, is extracted. Artemisinin is by far the most effective drug for malaria but Western society became aware of this compound only in the 1980s. And, it took almost two decades for the WHO to endorse its usage worldwide. Finally, the drug became an approved choice for the treatment of malaria in 2004. However, imagine how many lives were put in danger for all these years simply because the World Health Organization didn't view Artemisinin as a genuine treatment for malaria.

There are thousands of other natural herbal medicines that are effective in treating illness, but we are not familiar with them simply because modern medicine fails to acknowledge their efficacy.

Efficacy of Modern Medicine Questioned

The average American believes that modern medicine is constantly improving and medicines for new diseases are constantly invented by scientists. However, we often forget the fact that we seldom see a newspaper headline suggesting that a medicine for some disease that has haunted the human race for years was invented. AIDS and Cancer are good examples. These two diseases have been around for many decades, but we have yet to find a 'complete solution' for them.

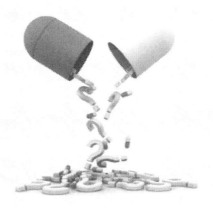

These are just examples, but there are thousands of illnesses that modern medicine is incapable of treating. Patients that are affected by such diseases often die in vain with the hope that medicine for their illness will be invented.

Even worse, trends in modern medicine suggest that most pharmaceutical companies are only interested in making money and they can go to any extent in pursuit of this goal. Their uncontrollable behavior, in many cases, causes serious health concerns for patients. Despite such problems, the manufacturers still go on to sell these drugs for several decades.

Prozac and Paxil are two examples of this. These drugs made their manufacturers millions of dollars before they were marred in massive controversy and lawsuits. The health consequences of these drugs were significant and evidences suggests that manufacturers ignored the downside of their drugs until various medical journals decided to reveal their true nature. Interestingly, in these cases the manufacturer is rarely charged with anything and walks free despite their drugs causing serious health problems or even death to thousands of innocent citizens, including children. [6]

In a nutshell, modern medicine doesn't live up to the expectations of its supporters. Most diseases are not completely cured with modern medicine. For many effective treatment programs found in modern medicine, a complement can be found in alternative medicine. Additionally, with advancements in science, it is much easier to verify the efficacy of herbs and other natural elements as treatments.

Scientists are finding it easier to understand the actual reasons behind the effectiveness of alternative treatment methods, and it is an undeniable truth that alternative medicine has fewer side effects compared to modern medicine.

Significance of Alternative Medicine

It is often assumed that the advocates of alternative medicine are the ones that practice it. Actually, there are notable figures in scientific history that understood its significance. Unfortunately, medical society and the media often view such opinions with skepticism. There are many examples of this: the most interesting one being the story of Dr. Linus Pauling, one of the only four people in the world to have won a Nobel price twice. Dr. Linus Pauling is also one of the only two people that have won a Nobel Prize for two different subjects.

He shocked the medical world by claiming that the major reason for most cardiovascular diseases is the deficiency of Vitamin C, a

---

[6] Web.Me. Accessed May 15, 2012.
http://web.me.com/stevescrutton/Banned_Pharma_Drugs/Prozac-Seroxat.html

claim that medical society simply ignored. Even worse, the mainstream media didn't pay enough attention to his claims. It would have been perfectly understandable if Dr. Pauling was simply a nobody without proven academic credentials or a history of treating people. Obviously, this was not the case here and this example shows how skewed the media is against alternative therapy.

Orthomolecular Medicine

Dr. Pauling introduced the concept of Orthomolecular Medicine to the world, one of the most successful alternative therapy methods introduced to the human race. The modern medical community took more than 3 decades to even acknowledge that perhaps Dr. Pauling could be right prior to studying it.

During his lifetime, Dr. Pauling treated several thousands of patients and successfully cured cardiovascular diseases. Despite this, most of his achievements were ignored by modern medicine and the media. It is difficult to call this pure coincidence, seeing that the medical industry is a multi-billion dollar behemoth controlled by a few pharmaceutical giants.

The media benefited from these companies in the form of advertisements and these companies had powerful purchasing power. This is something that no publication or broadcast venue wanted to ignore.

It is highly disappointing to notice that Dr. Pauling is the only person in the world that has a patented treatment method for cardiovascular diseases and he is the first person that suggested a working solution for the common cold. He advised heavy doses of Vitamin C to subdue the common cold but many laughed at his theory. Of course, it was later proven that a high intake of Vitamin C does subdue the common cold and a few other diseases.

Homeopathy – It's Not Just About Sugar

Homeopathy is a popular alternative therapy method, but if a patient claims that they had been cured by a homeopathic treatment people will either regard their illness as 'silly' or the person as exaggerating the benefits. Homeopathy is incredibly inexpensive and patients don't have to worry about spending their entire savings on treatments. Although insurance covers various types of treatments, it is difficult to claim insurance for an experimental treatment program. This is where an inexpensive alternative treatment method such as homeopathy has an advantage.

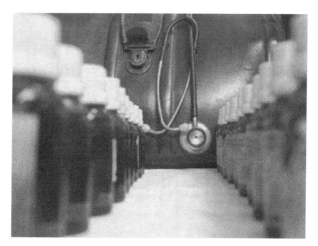

Homeopathy is also known for treatment programs with no side effects. A patient has nothing to lose by trying homeopathic treatment as it won't affect their health. Homeopathy is highly effective in treating infertility and there are many proven cases where homeopathic patients successfully conceived after many failed treatments from modern medicine.

Homeopathy believes that our body should be in harmony with nature and a typical treatment program urges you to keep a certain diet and live in a healthy atmosphere.

Chiropractic Treatment Method

Chiropractic is the second largest primary healthcare methodology in the world and the treatment philosophy focuses on health and the prevention of diseases. Chiropractic treatment focuses extensively on vascular and nutritional relationships, spinal biomechanics, musculoskeletal and neurological relationships. [7]

A chiropractic physician believes in the human body's unmatchable ability to cure itself from physical and emotional stress, trauma and similar disorders.

The human body is connected by three nervous systems including the central nervous system (brain and the spinal cord), peripheral nervous system and the autonomic nervous system. Science has proven that our nervous system is connected to all the tissues in the human body and any disorder in the central nervous system will create health problems in the human body.

It is hard to ignore the contributions of chiropractic medicine to modern science, especially includes a better understanding of the spinal cord and the central nervous system. A chiropractic practitioner starts his treatment by asking the health history of a patient and a physical examination is done after

---

[7] Think Quest. Accessed May 15, 2012.
http://library.thinkquest.org/24206/chiropractic.html

understanding the patient's health condition. Spinal manipulation, the most notable feature of chiropractic, is widely regarded as safe. However, Chiropractic Physicians utilize a breadth of techniques, methods and modalities in addition to manipulation in order to treat patients. Chiropractic physicians use what is known as the 'Triangle of Health' to help bring their patient's physiology into health and balance. This triangle of health consists of three sides, the structural, or physical, the bio-chemical, and the mental-emotional. When any one of these sides is affected, it also affects the other two sides of the triangle. This approach to good health by Chiropractic results in perfect balance within the human organism. Often, ailments are prevented from even arising due to the perfect balance of health that arises in all three sides of the triangle. [8]

How Is Chiropractic Treatment Done?

It is estimated that one in every four adults in the United States experience lower back pain. Although this is a startling statistic, modern medicine has failed to come up with long lasting remedies for this health problem. Most treatment methods for lower back pain in modern medicine are not only proven to be less effective but are also accompanied by many side effects. Chiropractic, on the other hand, has proven its efficacy in treating lower back pain and in many cases leads to the pain being gone completely.

The basic concepts of chiropractic medicine are:

- It is important to use human body's powerful, yet natural ability to heal when treating an illness.

---

[8] Wikipedia. Accessed May 15, 2012.
http://en.wikipedia.org/wiki/Chiropractic

- Bones, joints and muscles are closely intertwined and their natural harmony is very important for a healthy life.
- Chiropractic can bring back human body's natural balance.

The first step in starting a chiropractic treatment is taking the extra time to examine your body's condition. This is used to diagnose your problem and the treatment is determined after this.

The Significance of Alternative Therapy

As we have observed earlier, the majority of health disorders, including obesity and sleeping problems, that today's generation has to deal with is a result of changing lifestyles, diet and living conditions. This is something that supporters of modern medicine agree with. However, when it comes to alternative therapy and alternative health practices, they are resistant in admitting that alternative therapy has some benefits in treating 'modern-day' diseases.

Acid reflux disease is a good example for observing the benefits of alternative therapy. You can completely heal this disease with the help of diet and lifestyle changes but most patients still undergo expensive medical treatments that have serious side effects.[9] The advantage with alternative therapy for treating acid reflux disease is that you not only get rid of a health ailment that was haunting you, perhaps for a long time, but you can also improve your personal health dramatically. The

---

[9] Mayo Clinic. Accessed May 15, 2012.
http://www.mayoclinic.com/health/chiropractic-adjustment/MY01107/DSECTION=why-its-done

modern medical solution for acid reflux disease is not effective in providing long term relief. Moreover, overdoing the treatment will also give you other serious side effects. [10] Most chronic diseases are an immediate result of health and lifestyle changes and the best way to stay away from these disorders is practicing a healthy diet and lifestyle.

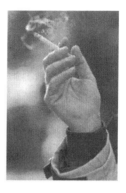

For instance, smokers and overweight people have a high probability of acquiring cardiovascular disease. By avoiding smoking and maintaining a healthy weight, you can dramatically reduce the chances of getting a chronic disorder.

However, modern medicine still insists on heavy medication once someone is diagnosed with such diseases, as opposed to suggesting serious lifestyle changes to the patient.

Nature has given us the enormous ability to fight several battles; famine is one among them. Our body can survive and perform many activities even if you are not getting food for many days. However, this enormous affinity for survival is not

---

[10] Web Medical Directory. Accessed May 15, 2012.
http://www.webmd.com/heartburn-gerd/treating-acid-reflux-disease-with-diet-lifestyle-changes

always a favorable one. Since food is plentiful for most of us, we are prone to store more fat with the wrong diet simply because our body will keep the excess food to fight a famine that will never come.

Researchers suggest that people from Asia, Latin America and Africa are more prone to obesity with diet changes as their genes have a better ability to fight hunger. The modern diet and lifestyle put them at the risk of being overweight as they would probably never experience a food crisis. [11]

Examples from the Developing World

You can see many examples from the developing world that support this argument. Populations in South East Asia, India and China are benefiting heavily from globalization. Several multinational companies are setting up their offices in these locations. These countries are now exposed to the working habits of the developed world, which fetches them much better income than the traditional job opportunities they had been used to.

The new generation in the developing world is now seeking education that will get them placed in these multinational companies and the per capita income and GDP of countries that welcomed globalization is steadily going up. It is believed that China is going to be world's largest economy by 2050.

Despite such a promising economic boom in these countries, they are facing a serious problem. A good number of young

---

[11] Web Medical Directory. Accessed May 15, 2012.
http://www.webmd.com/heartburn-gerd/treating-acid-reflux-disease-with-diet-lifestyle-changes

individuals in these nations – individuals who are supposed to be the stepping stones of success for these countries – are going through serious health problems such as anxiety, stress, obesity and heart problems.

Governments in these countries are worried because the young generation that is supposed to lead these countries to their long desired success is falling ill much before their elders. This young generation has a much wider waistline than most of their ancestors and heart attacks are no longer a foreign word for them. As a matter of fact, heart diseases and cardiac arrests are so common among this young generation that such incidents rarely attract any attention from their colleagues apart from the obvious sympathy.

Supporters of alternative medicine in these countries argue that modern medicine has a role to play in spoiling the health of their new generation, a claim that the governments in these countries ignored for very long. With constant interferences from the World Health Organization and United Nations, these countries have worked hard to establish competent modern medicine facilities in their cities. These countries also make sure that the vaccinations and drugs suggested by the WHO are available in their smaller cities as well.

A very disappointing example is India, the home of Ayurveda. Although Ayurveda is proven to be a powerful treatment method and the medicinal values of several herbs are scientifically known, the Indian government paid very little attention to the promotion of Ayurvedic treatment in the country. Some of the leading Ayurvedic treatment facilities in India such as Kottackal Arya Vaidya Shala are private treatment facilities, and the government support these facilities receive is negligible.

An immediate effect of government negligence is Ayurvedic treatment becoming very expensive. Today, most Indians can't afford traditional Ayurvedic treatments without spending a hefty sum of money. Despite its lateness of recognition, the good news is that Indian government is slowly realizing the importance of incorporating Ayurvedic treatments into mainstream medical facilities. Many government initiatives are already taken in its favor.

How Can Alternative Medicine Help You Live Longer?

It goes without saying that modern medicine is an absolute failure in treating most modern diseases, which are a direct result of changing lifestyles, eating habits and sleep problems. The problem with modern medicine is that it has limited exposure to sensitive areas such as diet and obesity. Modern medicine tries to address most health ailments with drugs despite the fact that, in most cases, today's patients need only a minor change in their day-to-day routine.

It is surprising to see that the medical industry is reluctant to admit that treatments without chemical drugs can work in treating cardiovascular disease and many physical ailments. The traditional medicine industry, instead of adopting a critical view of drugs, heavily depends on chemical substances to address most problems. The biggest downside of this approach is the side effects of these drugs.

With the traditional medical approach, it is nearly impossible for a patient to completely resolve a problem without any side effects. In other words, a health condition that is solved or treated with chemical substances can leave you with lifelong side effects. Most of us are looking for a treatment method that will solve our problems forever and help us lead a healthy life. Unfortunately, modern medicine doesn't sound like the answer for this desire.

Alternative medicine, on the other hand, has thousands of years of experience in working on health problems with diet changes, therapy and nutritional food supply. Alternative medicine believes in the body's ability to heal itself and at best, it offers the human body a helping hand in fighting unexpected problems.

An alternative treatment procedure doesn't consist of any chemical drugs. Most herbs or substances, if any are used for treatment, are derived from plant or animal sources that pose no serious threat to a human body. Appreciating the importance of a healthy diet is the biggest positive point of alternative medicine.

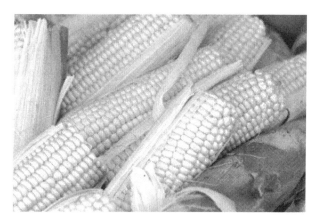

At the end of an alternative treatment procedure, a patient is not only free from any diseases but they also enjoy better health overall: a direct result of the dietary and lifestyle changes that they had to undergo during treatment.

Alternative Therapy in a Nutshell

Compared to modern medicine, alternative therapy has several advantages and it is evident that following an alternative medical lifestyle will reduce your body's drug dependency. By following a healthy lifestyle, you will improve your overall health. People that follow alternative medical treatment usually maintains better physique (provided that they are adhering to the treatment methods strictly) and are less prone to serious heart disorders. By staying away from harmful chemical drugs, they are much less exposed to many health disorders that are a direct result of medical drug usage.

Alternative therapy also has many distinct advantages from a financial point of view. Diagnosis and treatment is usually very inexpensive in alternative therapy.

If everybody decides to follow an alternative therapy lifestyle, governments can dramatically reduce their spending on health budgets. If governments are taking serious initiatives to promote alternative therapy, several billion of dollars spent on chemical drugs can be saved. The obvious downside of such an initiative is that the ever growing drug industry will come to a halt and these companies are not going to appreciate it.

With the purchasing power of large multinational companies in control of politics and media in many countries, they are capable of preventing governments from taking drastic measures against the medical drug industry. The only solution for the promotion of alternative medicine is creating awareness in patients so that they are capable of choosing between right and wrong.

What Every Woman Must Know

Chapter 2:

Unique Health Problems Connected With Female Physiology

Many people don't realize just how unique some problems that women suffer from actually are. Besides this, many health problems also affect a woman far more seriously than they affect men in general. One could link these differences to the essential differences between male and female physiology.

Many medical techniques don't really focus on this essential difference, leading to serious drawbacks in the way these systems (and especially traditional allopathic medicine) treat women's health problems. Some branches of alternative medicine recognize the essential difference between male and female physiology.[12] Chiropractic, for example, is one of the medical systems that has always focused on and applied itself to treating the unique health issues that women can suffer from.

Besides the essential uniqueness of women's problems, it has also been found that women are more aware of their bodies, and are more ready to seek help if they perceive a problem. As

---

[12] Holistic Healing. Accessed May 15, 2012.http://www.holistic-mindbody-healing.com/allopathic-medicine.html

a matter of fact, more women than men are found to rely upon effective systems of alternative medicine, such as Chiropractic.

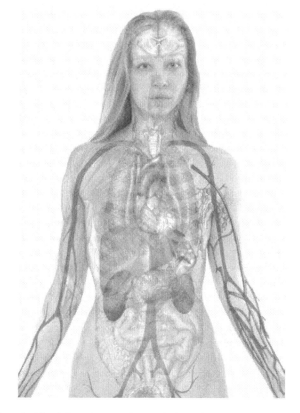

Female Physiology is complex and gives rise to a unique set of ailments and issues

Unique issues arise from a unique structure

Many unique health problems in women have their root in the fact that the female body is designed around the bearing of children. Pregnancy can cause or affect many health issues, as can the menstrual cycle. Causes related to these things can result in chronic pain in the pelvic region, as well as pain when a woman is menstruating. There are also chemical and mental or emotional problems that can arise from these issues.

As a woman grows older, she is also more likely than a man to experience certain ailments.[13] Alzheimer's is a prime example of this, but osteoporosis is also an issue that a majority of women will suffer from without medical intervention. With Alzheimer's, a person's mind and memory are seriously affected, while osteoporosis can weaken the bones to an extent that can be life-threatening.

Women are also a great deal more likely to suffer from chronic headaches – an issue which, if less serious than the two conditions mentioned before it, is nevertheless capable of seriously detracting from a person's quality of life. Arthritis is also a condition that is between two to three times more likely to affect a woman than a man. We'll be discussing the unique health problems that can affect a woman in more detail in the course of this chapter.

The essential differences between male and female physiology...

While most of the common characteristic differences between men and women are well known, many people don't realize that these differences extend, in many cases, to the very functioning of the organs. These differences in the functioning of the organs can actually affect the way in which the body works.

---

[13] Canadian Women's Health Network. Accessed May 15, 2012. http://www.cwhn.ca/en/node/42145

Some examples of physiological differences between men and women...

For example, there are considerable differences in lung capacity in men and women, with the advantage in function being entirely on the side of the male. This can limit the capacity for exercise in a woman (as compared to a man). This difference becomes especially important as a woman ages. The structure of women's brains also differs to some extent from that of a man's, resulting from the effects of gonadal hormones when in the fetal stages of development.

The heart also differs in male and female physiology, with the female heart having a considerably smaller left ventricle. This ensures that considerable more blood is propelled through the cardiovascular system per beat of the heart.

However, there are even more integral differences in the functioning of the cardiovascular system in men and women.[14] For example, women have a far lower electrocardiogram Q-T interval. This means that certain life-threatening conditions of the heart, such as arrhythmia, can be far more serious for women than for men.

These are just a few examples. In reality, the differences between the physiology of men and women are far more deep-set. Everything from lipid metabolism to the regulation of fluids within the body as well as the electrolyte balance is affected by these differences.

---

[14] NCBI. Accessed May 15, 2012.
http://www.ncbi.nlm.nih.gov/pubmed/17327577

The bottom line is that any medical practitioner needs to take these crucial differences into account when treating a woman, but unfortunately few medical practitioners, especially in traditional western medicine, do.

Women's health in America:

The simple fact is that women's special needs are rarely considered when they consult a traditional western practitioner. This is especially true in America, and this means that the standard of care for women is a good deal lower than it should be.

A considerable percentage of women go through life suffering some level of discomfort or pain caused by factors that are unique to the female physiology.

These factors can result in anything from chronic pelvic or back pain to crucial issues like osteoporosis, which can be crippling to a woman later in life.

The best way to view the factors that affect a woman's health is the Chiropractic way. Chiropractic looks at human health as being affected by a triangle of factors. Each side of the triangle represents one crucial facet of human health, and all the sides support each other.

If one side of the triangle is lacking, the other sides of the triangle are affected as well. The three sides of this 'health triangle', according to Chiropractic, are the structural, the chemical, and the mental-emotional. We will now take a look at what problems women in America face in each of the above areas...

Structural issues:

Many factors influence upper back pain in women, but some common causes are incorrect posture or a chronic straining of the muscles of the upper back.

However, in women, other factors can also cause upper back pain.

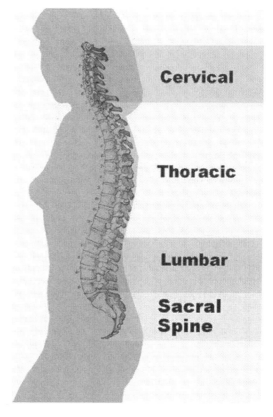

For example, arthritis, which women are up to three times more likely to suffer from, is a common cause of upper back pain.

Inflammation caused by this condition can affect the vertebrae of the spine, and cause considerable discomfort as well as seriously interfere with a person's ability to lead a normal life. Another factor that can cause upper back pain in women is Osteoporosis, which causes a serious lack of density in the bones, sometimes resulting in hairline fractures. Often enough, Osteoporosis does not show until post-menopause, when it can have serious consequences. Since Osteoporosis is actually a result of a loss of calcium content in the body all through one's life, it can be countered by consulting with a specialist in preventive medicine, such as Chiropractic, who can take steps to prevent the condition from ever arising. Another related condition that can be prevented by the right care is Osteoarthritis, which a considerable percentage of older women are likely to suffer from.

Lower back pain:

Many of the factors that cause upper back pain also cause pain in the lower back. However, the lower back carries most of the weight of the upper torso, and is far more prone to injuries of various kinds. Also, there are factors unique to female physiology that can result in lower back pain. Pregnancy, for example, can result in lower back pain at various stages ranging from early in the term to the late stages. Pregnancy can even result in lower back pain post-partum. This is because the weight of the baby can place a considerable strain upon the spine. If other ailments, such as incipient arthritis or a herniated disc, also occur at the same time the lower back pain can become a most serious condition. Various ailments can also result in lower back pain, and treating such pain must also include treatment of the underlying condition. Some of these problems include infections of the intestine or the bladder, or even conditions that affect the sexual organs in women. Some kinds of cancer can also cause lower back pain, and it is crucial to consult a qualified practitioner at the earliest possible opportunity if you suffer from chronic lower back pain.

Headaches:

Headaches are certainly a structural issue that women suffer from a great deal more frequently than men. Three quarters of those who suffer from chronic headaches in America are women.[15] It might be surprising to know that most of these women are below the age of forty and have to balance the demands of a career with their commitments to the home. This makes the headaches these women suffer from a debilitating condition. But why are those who suffer from headaches so predominantly female? Some researchers believe that migraine headaches might well be a side effect of hormones like estrogen. This is supported by the fact that headaches affect both females and males to about the same extent when they are children, and only tend to affect women more after they attain puberty. There seems to be a definite connection between the menstrual cycle and the incidence of chronic headaches as well. There is certain evidence to support the fact that women who suffer from chronic migraines might see an increase in the number or intensity of these symptoms during pregnancy. It has also been observed that an increase in chronic headaches occurs as a woman nears menopause.

---

[15] Scientific American. Accessed May 15, 2012. http://www.scientificamerican.com/article.cfm?id=why-women-report-being-in

Sport injuries

Many injuries are caused in the course of training for various sports, because the muscles and ligaments are placed under much stress. Women are especially prone to some injuries, such as tears of the anterior cruciate ligaments. This sort of injury is usually caused either by a sharp injury or heavy impact, or by regularly applying twisting stress to the joint.

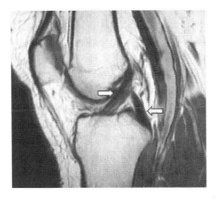

Stress upon the cruciate ligaments

A serious level of disability results from tearing the anterior cruciate ligaments. Another injury that is known to affect female athletes more than men is shin splints. The reason why this injury is more prevalent in female athletes than in men is not completely clear at this time, but it is known that not only are women more prone to this sort of injury, but they are more than three times likely to suffer complications as a result of it. Plantar Fasciitis, which affects a band of connective tissue in the foot, is also common among female athletes. A person suffering from Plantar Fasciitis may have problems in moving the foot because of the condition. It is postulated that women suffer from this condition to a greater extent than men because the center of gravity in their bodies is lower. [16]

Chronic pain

Chronic pain is also an issue that a large number of women suffer from, and the reasons why have intrigued researchers for decades. Many researchers believe that the female experience of pain is linked to hormones like estrogen, which seem to intensify the sensations of pain. The pain processing areas in women's brains may also function differently from those of men. It has been found that certain pain suppressing medications work differently for men and women, with some of the medications being more effective for women than for men and vice versa. All this points to the fact that men and women process the sensations of pain differently. There is also evidence that the experience of pain in the different sexes might be linked to genetics, with a greater sensitivity to pain in women descending through the genes. Then again, women experience processes like menstruation, which place a considerable strain upon the body and which can add to their experience of pain. However, there is some evidence that men might quite simply be suppressing their pain or at least avoiding reporting it, due to societal pressure upon men to do so.

---

[16] Beth Israel Deaconess Medical Center. Accessed May 15, 2012. http://www.bidmc.org/YourHealth/HealthNotes/BonesandJoints/SportsInjuriesandPrevention/WomenandSportsInjuries.aspx

Chemical health issues that affect American women today

Anything that disrupts the chemical functioning of the body can have serious consequences for health, and women are more prone to chemical imbalances than men because their biochemical makeup is more subtle and more easily upset. The chemical balance in a woman's body can be upset by various factors, including taking in too much highly processed junk food, as well as by drinking too much coffee. Smoking and alcohol are also serious risk factors because these things seem to affect women more seriously than they do men. For example, if we examine a man and a woman of exactly the same weight, we find that it takes thirty percent less alcohol to make the woman drunk. This is because male bodies produce a protective enzyme that breaks down up to thirty percent of ingested alcohol. This is probably a protective measure developed by men over centuries of ingesting alcohol in large quantities. Women, perhaps lacking a similar evolution, also lack the defenses against alcohol created by that evolution. Nutrition can also be a serious issue affecting the chemical balance in a woman. Weight loss fads can result in a massive depletion of essential nutrients in the body, with serious consequences.

Weight loss issues that cause chemical imbalances

A considerable section of the female population of the United States has a problem with excess, unhealthy weight. A great many factors can cause this, but female physiology is one of the reasons why so many American women struggle with excess weight as they grow older. Generally speaking, most women have a slower metabolism than men, and a greater percentage of body fat. What this translates into is a tendency to put on weight. With a slower metabolism, it's harder to lose weight once you put it on. These days a good many specialists are advising women to train with weights, because this adds to the lean muscle in their physical makeup and ups their metabolism. But more factors than merely a slower metabolism can be at the root of excessive weight gain in a woman. One such factor is polycystic ovarian syndrome, which can result in hormonal imbalances within the body that can make it extremely difficult for a woman to lose weight. A thyroid condition can also create a chemical imbalance within the body that can make it very easy to put on weight, and hard to lose those excess pounds. If you suffer from an underlying condition that is causing you to put on excess weight, then treating that underlying condition might be crucial.

Excessive fatigue

Excessive fatigue is another problem that many American women suffer from today. Chronic fatigue can sometimes be addressed by simply making alterations in one's lifestyle. Our lifestyle today is one that is highly conducive to overwork, insomnia and stress. Moreover, it is one that human physiology, and especially the female physiology, was never evolved for. Changing one's lifestyle choices around to show a bit more consideration towards one's body can result in a significant reduction in levels of chronic fatigue. Even so, not all cases of chronic fatigue can be addressed in this way. It is observed that in about one in every five cases of chronic fatigue among women, the underlying cause of the fatigue was *not* the woman's lifestyle but rather a physical illness.

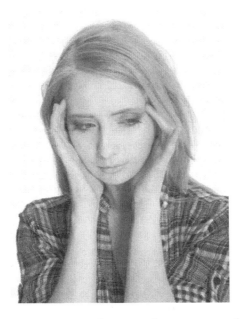

There are a great many ailments that can result in chronic fatigue, and treating them, rather than merely trying to address the fatigue itself, is all important if the patient is to experience relief. Various causes of fatigue can range from anemia, which is a lack of iron in the body, to poor diet and nutrition. Other causes of fatigue can include an underactive thyroid gland, a urinary tract infection, or even sleep apnea - in which a patient's natural sleep cycle is disrupted leading to insufficient rest.

Lifestyle and dietary choices

The lifestyle and dietary choices a woman makes can have a profound impact on her health.[17] Lifestyle choices can result in

---

[17] LiveStrong.com. Accessed May 15, 2012.
http://www.livestrong.com/healthy-diet-plan/

excessive fatigue and a variety of stress related conditions. Often enough in today's world, a person finds themselves forced to work far beyond their capacity, perhaps with looming 'deadlines' in the background. Levels of stress can be even higher if there is a personal stake in the matter, such as a person is running their own business. Whatever the circumstances, such high levels of fatigue and stress are anything but desirable. When you add incorrect nutrition to this, the situation becomes very serious indeed. Often enough, a person may simply not have the time to eat correctly, and may rely on junk food to get them through the day. While this might be barely acceptable as a short term dietary strategy, it is completely unacceptable in the long term and can cause serious damage to health. A result of a combination of the above factors can result in heart problems, diabetes, arteriosclerosis, kidney issues, and a host of other physical problems as the body is pushed beyond its limits and its chemical balance is disrupted. As a result of the lifestyle of the overstressed and overworked women of today, mental problems like depression are also becoming very common.

Constipation

Constipation in women is usually caused when a woman doesn't take in enough fluids. It can happen in the course of the day that a person just doesn't feel thirsty. This can be due to a chemical imbalance in the body that results in a person not feeling thirsty even though the body needs water. Whatever the cause, not taking in enough fluid daily can result in constipation as the body attempts to absorb water from ingested food instead. A lack of fiber can also lead to increasing levels of constipation. While much of this is fairly well known, many people do not know that a lack of physical activity and exercise can also contribute to constipation. Bowel movement seems to be keyed to physical activity, and not doing sufficient exercise can cause extreme irregularity. Staying active physically can usually go a long way towards preventing constipation, in conjunction with other factors like taking in enough fluids and fiber. Remember that physical exercise affects the entire body, not merely the muscles used in the course of your activity. Regular and spirited physical exercise has a salutary effect not only upon the internal organs, but also on the mental and emotional components as well.

General toxicity within the body

While there are all sorts of methods advocated to detoxify the body, perhaps the best method of all is to avoid toxicity in the first place. In other words, a little prevention is preferable to even the best cure. There are more sources of toxins in your environment than you might think. Health and beauty products can be a source of toxins, as can various cleaning agents used around the house. There's paint and glues and the various kinds of varnishes, as well as gasoline. And of course there are pesticides and fertilizers that we might inadvertently take in along with our food. Any or all of these substances can contribute to general toxicity in a woman's body. Coffee is a prime offender because the least possible care is taken when growing it to avoid harmful pesticides. The roasting process that it is subjected to also leaves oils that can turn rancid and harmful with great rapidity. Worse, it is also a diuretic. Beauty products are also contributors to toxicity, because they frequently contain endocrine disruptors as well as substances that can cause congestion in the liver. Artificial sweeteners should also be avoided since the body can break them down into harmful neurotoxins. Finally, it goes without saying that smoking and alcohol can contribute massively to toxicity within the body.

Dehydration

With a major percentage of the body consisting of water, dehydration can be a far more serious condition than most people might think. A considerable percentage of working women in America suffer from dehydration, which can directly be linked to a busy lifestyle in which people simply do not take in enough water, but also to the prevalence in our culture of various artificial drinks that simply don't do as much as water towards rehydrating the body. Remember that symptoms of dehydration in women can often manifest themselves as something other than simple thirst. Often enough, a woman who is dehydrated will experience an all-encompassing tiredness and fatigue, despite getting enough rest at night. This may be accompanied by dizziness as well as by irritability and headaches. If you're suffering from any of these symptoms, you should consider that they might be caused by your body simply not getting enough water. Often enough, rehydrating the body by taking in enough pure and unpolluted water can result in a near miraculous recession of these symptoms. Remember that chronic dehydration can be extremely dangerous, placing a severe strain on the kidneys and liver and also causing unhealthy weight gain.

Heavy metal toxicity

Heavy metal toxicity can seriously disrupt the chemical balance in a woman's body, yet this is a problem that an increasing number of women in the United States suffer from. As a matter of fact, quite a few heavy metals are necessary and indeed even beneficial to the body. However, these are needed by the body in small quantities. Iron is a very good example of this, with the body's entire oxygen-transport mechanism being based on iron. However, even iron can be extremely harmful if ingested in far greater quantities than the body needs. Some of the heavy metals that contaminate our environment (and our bodies) today include lead and arsenic, as well as cadmium and mercury. Any and all of these elements can cause serious issues within the body. Arsenic can enter the body by eating shellfish that originated in contaminated zones of water. Paint and some fungicides can also be sources of arsenic, which is why it is best to source your vegetables from organic farms that do not use these products. Lead is another extremely dangerous element that at one time was used heavily in pipes and as paint in houses. Fortunately, the use of lead for these purposes has dropped off in recent years. Nevertheless, caution is necessary, especially if you happen to live in a house or apartment that was built in the 1970s. Mercury can be found in bottom feeding fish, in thermometers, and in children's vaccines.

Allergies

Anyone who keeps up with the news knows that allergies seem to be on the increase in America and indeed in all developed countries. The root cause of this is uncertain, but some studies point to excessive hygiene. For example, a study conducted a few years ago found that children who lived in a more natural country environment, rather than in a city, were a lot less likely to develop common allergies, such as the allergy to peanuts or an allergy to cats. [18]Those who lived in a more 'sanitary' (that is, a less natural) environment in which they did not come into

---

[18] Allergic Living. Accessed May 15, 2012.
http://allergicliving.com/index.php/2010/11/20/allergies-why-so-many-now/?page=3

contact with these so-called allergic triggers at an early age were several times more likely to develop allergies. Studies have also found that children who are part of a large family are less likely to develop allergies than single children, presumably because children in large families are exposed to each other. Similarly, children who come into contact with pets and farm animals at a young age are several times less likely to develop allergies. Women have traditionally been less susceptible to allergies than men. However, this trend seems to be changing, with women showing a distinct tendency to cat allergies and hay fever, as well as to many 'technological' triggers.

Asthma

Is there a difference in how asthma affects men and women? Recent research shows that this might well be the case, with a larger percentage of women than men developing symptoms of asthma after puberty. It has been observed that pregnancy, for example, can increase the severity of asthma attacks. Many medical specialists postulate that certain female hormones might well increase the severity of the symptoms of asthma. Estrogen is thought to be a particular cause of this, though considerable clinical research needs to be conducted in this area.

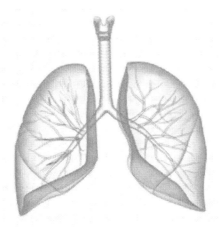

The human lungs

The basic differences between male and female physiology could also be said to be the reason why women seem to experience asthma attacks with greater severity. The lungs in women are considerably smaller than those of men, and the bronchial tubes might also tend to be narrower. This of course usually tends to increase the severity of attacks in asthmatic women. There may also be genetic influences at work here, but the reasons why women experience asthma in more serious forms than men remain largely unexplained. Some medical researchers believe that women simply spend more time in the home, and that the home environment is a source of many concentrated allergens.

Mental and emotional issues that American women suffer from today

Over a quarter of the female population in America today suffers from one mental and emotional issue or another.[19] In terms of numbers, that amounts to nearly thirty million women. Remember that we are talking only about diagnosed cases, and thus undiagnosed cases may well be far more in number. For example, two times as many American women will experience depression in the course of their lives than men. Twice as many women as men in America suffer from various phobias and anxiety, as well as from various other issues like obsessive-compulsive disorder. Other issues that American women suffer from are panic disorder, post-traumatic stress and eating disorders. Eating disorders are especially prevalent among the female sections of the population. For example, the vast majority of anorexia sufferers are female. Females also tend to be binge eaters, with sixty five percent of cases of this disorder being women. Part of the reason why there is such a predominance of women in cases of depression and anxiety is due to the effect of fluctuations in the levels of female hormones. Schizophrenic women suffer especially severe attacks during their menstrual cycles. Various other factors also contribute to mental and emotional conditions in women, so we'll examine the most common of these in more detail.

---

[19] National Institute of Mental Health. Accessed May 15, 2012. http://wwwapps.nimh.nih.gov/health/publications/the-numbers-count-mental-disorders-in-america.shtml

Depression

The numbers indicate that women have a greater susceptibility to depression than men. Not only is this so, but it has been observed that often enough the very causes of depression in men and women differ, as do the symptoms that they suffer from. Depression among women in America is caused by a great many factors. Female hormones play a part, as discussed in the earlier paragraph, but stress, and social and economic pressures also play a major role as causes of depression.

There are many symptoms of depression, but if a woman chronically feels sad or guilty or even tired, she may be suffering from depression. Other signs of being depressed include losing interest in activities that you used to enjoy. Suicidal thoughts are also an obvious sign of depression, but a more subtle one may be disrupted sleep patterns. Beware of either insomnia (an inability to sleep) or a tendency to sleep too much – either is a sign of depression. The same applies to appetite – a loss of appetite or a tendency to eat too much both point to possible depression. People who are depressed also might have problems concentrating on anything, and may feel a general sense of lassitude and fatigue.

Post-partum depression:

A considerable percentage of new mothers will develop post-partum depression: a depression that occurs just after the term of pregnancy is over and the baby is born. The exact causes of this are uncertain, but it is postulated that this sort of depression is caused by complex chemical imbalances in a woman's body post-partum. Remember that this is a time when a woman's body is undergoing complex changes. Levels of estrogen are low, and this can cause mood swings and depression. At around this time thyroid levels also plummet. Both of these factors result in depression and can also result in increased levels of fatigue. These factors can lead to even greater levels of depression in a sort of vicious circle. Post-partum depression is not to be underestimated, as women suffering from this condition have actually committed extreme acts of violence against themselves, and sometimes even against their children. Besides hormonal imbalances, another cause of post-partum depression is that many women feel unattractive in the period just after child-birth. Of course, the stress and sleepless nights that come with the care of a newborn child can be a major cause of feelings of excessive fatigue that can easily turn into depression.

Anxiety

More and more women in America today are seeking help for anxiety-related issues. Though these issues affect both men and women, women suffer from anxiety related ailments twice as often as men. This is something that can seriously affect the quality of life of a woman. A woman who suffers from anxiety and related issues is likely to make serious lifestyle changes in an effort to reduce her levels of anxiety – this can include shifting to a lower paying job, which might bring in less money but be less stressful. It can also affect a woman's social life, because anxiety may cause her to limit her social interactions. Various different factors can trigger anxiety in women such as hormonal imbalances, which can include unnaturally low levels of the hormones progesterone and estrogen. A severe traumatic experience in the past can also cause recurring anxiety attacks, as can regular insomnia, a chemical imbalance in the body, or levels of chronic stress or fatigue. Genes have also been seen to play a role in how likely a woman is to suffer from anxiety attacks. If a woman suffers from anxiety attacks, it is crucial that she seek help, as the attacks tend to escalate in intensity if left untreated.

Bipolar Disorder

In bipolar disorder, a person's mood tends to swing between extremes of euphoria and depression. Bipolar disorder affects men and women quite differently, in that women tend to have more depressing episodes than episodes of euphoria. Of course, hormonal changes in a woman tend to increase the symptoms of this disorder. There are studies that indicate that menopause in older women might actually trigger the onset of bipolar disorder. Women suffering from severe PMS (premenstrual syndrome) can also experience the onset of bipolar disorder. As a matter of fact, it has been observed that a woman who is being treated for bipolar disorder can actually show lowered levels of PMS as well, clearly illustrating the connection between the causes and effects of these two disorders. Bipolar disorder can manifest itself in the greatest intensity during pregnancy and after the term is complete. If a woman already suffering from bipolar disorder becomes pregnant, it is far more likely that the disorder will take a serious turn after the birth of her child. Similarly, a woman who has been treated for bi-polar disorder is more likely to experience a relapse during pregnancy or after the birth of a child.

Various emotional issues that women in America suffer from...

One of the reasons women frequently suffer from emotional issues is hormonal flux. The levels of certain hormones change continuously in the course of a woman's life, and this can have an impact on her mental state. This may or may not be additionally influenced by various factors and stresses in her life, but the simple fact is that a woman who experiences no negative factors in her life can still have emotional issues solely due to hormonal flux. Generally speaking, Premenstrual syndrome, or PMS, can be one of the results of this hormonal flux, while depression can also be a resulting factor especially during or after pregnancy. Menopause syndrome is also a hormone-related issue that can affect older women. Besides this, hormonal flux can also result in anxiety attacks, especially if there is a traumatic event in a woman's past. Please note that traumatic in this sense need not be a large disaster or even a violent event in the past, but merely an event that the woman found traumatic. Symptoms of emotional distress include disrupted sleep patterns, low energy levels, and chronic feelings of sadness.

Emotional stress

More American women than ever suffer from stress related ailments these days, and it's quite plain why this is so. There is a very clearly defined idea in society as to what a woman's responsibilities in a home are, and this social idea forces women into trying to handle the pressures of running a home and (in a working woman) the pressures of a workplace. This is quite simply too much stress for the human psyche to handle, and results in a large percentage of women suffering from the effects of emotional stress. What we're discussing here is actually a best-case scenario. A woman with a perfectly stable home environment and merely reasonable pressures at work is still subjected to far higher levels of stress than are acceptable. If, on the other hand, the home environment is not stable, with frequent arguments with her spouse, and problems with her children, levels of stress can reach extremely dangerous levels. This might be accentuated by extreme pressures at work, something that is especially true in these times when companies try to extract the maximum possible out of their workers. Hormonal imbalances can combine with these unnaturally high levels of environmental stress with disastrous effects.

Worry

People worry about lots of things in life, and a certain amount of worry is perfectly natural. Problems occur, though, if it's allowed to get out of hand, when it can result in elevated levels of stress and anxiety, both of which can develop into more serious problems and issues. At the beginning of this chapter we talked about the chiropractic view of health as a triangle in which each side, the physical, the chemical, and the mental-emotional, supports the others. When you look at health from that point of view, excessive worry can be disastrous because it can result in mental and emotional issues that can become so serious that they can affect the other aspects of the health triangle. As a result, you can see people suffering from serious stress and anxiety disorders developing physical ailments, including heart disease, and perhaps even certain kinds of cancer. Yes, it is actually possible to worry oneself into illness, which is why it's important to keep the issues that one worries about in life under reasonable control. So what are the things that women worry about most?

Finances

In the uncertain economic climate of these modern times, it's inevitable that a woman should worry about money. The real focus of many women is family, but money is seen as a means to maintaining a family, and financial problems can affect a woman's mind perhaps more than any other issue. These financial worries can range from worry about a current situation to worries about the future, including issues like providing for the education of children.

Work

Work is an issue that women worry about, both in and of itself, and also because it directly impacts finances in the home. However, stresses generated in the workplace can also impact a woman's personal life and space, creating additional stresses at home.

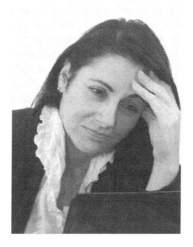

Women also tend to worry about how well they're doing things, about whether they're performing well enough both in the spheres of work and the home. Some women can feel a sense of inadequacy if one of these spheres dominates the other. For example, a woman might feel stressed if her job demands time that she feels she should be spending with her family, and vice versa.

Health

Health is another issue that women tend to worry over. Women often study nutrition and take up exercise not merely to maintain their appearance, but also to maintain good health. One might say that women seem to be more naturally health conscious than men. However, this consciousness of health can also translate into worry. Keeping fit and taking vitamins, as well as being alert for the symptoms of an ailment are all positive tendencies, but it is essential to not let these things escalate into paranoia.

Family

Children can cause a lot of worry to both parents, but especially to a woman. As a matter of fact, a woman can worry about children even before she's pregnant or before they are born. Women who've never had children can worry about whether they are fertile. If they are past thirty, they can worry about whether increasing age will interfere with their ability to have children. Then, of course, there are the usual worries that a woman experiences during pregnancy. Caring for children has its own rather obvious worries and concerns.

Time schedules

With all the demands upon a woman's time, a major source of worry for a woman can simply be how she is to fit in all the things that seem to need doing in the course of a day. This worry can become a paranoia, or at the very least, an obsession.

Some kinds of obsessive-compulsive disorder have their roots in this simple worry.

Age

Aging is certainly a factor that women worry about. With the emphasis that many modern societies place upon a woman's looks, it's no wonder that the worry of losing those looks to age is a potent one. Instead of working to maintain their overall health, women become focused upon purely external appearances, often using potentially harmful plastic surgery and heavy make up to disguise the effects of age.

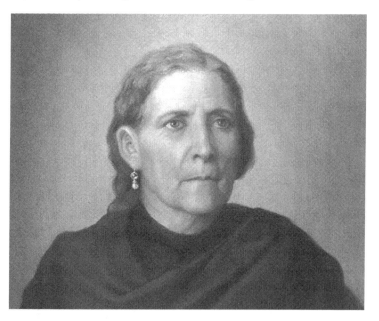

Appearance

Our society tends to brainwash women into being obsessed with their appearance. Billboards depict women selling everything from toothbrushes to handbags to jewelry and beyond. This can make women obsessed with their appearance, since there seems to be a subtle pressure in society for them to be that way. Whatever the reasons, this is something that women truly worry about. A woman may worry about whether she's too thin or whether she's putting on too much weight. As she gets older she may worry about whether she's losing her looks. None of these worries are particularly threatening, but they can be if they are allowed to get out of hand.

Weight gain

There are many subtle reasons why a woman might suddenly start to gain weight. These reasons can range from the purely physical to the biochemical and even have their roots in emotional causes. Diet and nutrition is a subject that can fill a whole book in itself, so we won't go into it in detail here. Suffice it to say that modern society forces people to accept a diet high in cereals and carbohydrates, and low in many essential nutrients. This is a diet that the human body was never evolved for. The result of such a diet can go beyond unhealthy weight gain to genuine malnutrition. Knowing what to eat can be crucial to maintaining one's health. Exercise is another component of unhealthy weight gain. All too often people in modern societies lead an extremely sedentary life, and by this lack of exercise they deny their bodies a chance for good health that is so easy to reach for. Even a minimum of exercise is so beneficial, yet often enough people will not reach even for that bare minimum. Women can also eat too much as a response to emotional issues or depression. There is actually a biochemical reason for this, as overindulgence in foods that contain carbohydrates can release serotonin within the body. This can calm the mind, and so it's no surprise that women can sometimes see eating as a plausible escape from their emotional issues. The price of this particular escape is, of course, excess weight.

Thyroid problems in women

Problems with the thyroid gland, and especially hypothyroidism, are very common in women.[20] Some of the most common symptoms of this are increased lethargy and fatigue. Remember that the thyroid gland is the body's mechanism for regulating metabolism. When it malfunctions, extreme fatigue is generally the first symptom. If one suffers fatigue despite having an undisturbed and deep sleep every night, a problem with the thyroid is plausibly to blame. Another sign of hypothyroidism is the inability to tolerate cold. Since the body's metabolism is lowered, it seems to lose the ability to warm itself effectively, and you may feel cold at temperatures that other people are perfectly comfortable with. Constipation can have many causes, of course, but it is also a symptom of hypothyroidism. If it appears in conjunction with the other symptoms, constipation can certainly be taken as an indicator of the condition. Other symptoms can include pain in the muscles, problems with the hair or the skin, and a sudden and unexplained increase in weight. Any problem with the thyroid is a potentially serious condition, and can have long term consequences. A person who experiences any or all of the above symptoms should consult a medical practitioner at once.

---

[20] E-Medicine Health. Accessed May 15, 2012.
http://www.emedicinehealth.com/thyroid_problems/article_em.htm

Adrenal insufficiency syndrome

The adrenal glands provide for a response to stress as well as regulating many other crucial aspects of bodily function, including controlling electrolyte and fluid content within the body. It goes without saying that a malfunction of the adrenal glands can have serious consequences. There is some evidence that women are more effected by conditions that affect the adrenal gland than men. Symptoms of adrenal deficiency may include weight loss, fatigue and a general weakness in the muscles. These symptoms are chronic in cases of adrenal deficiency, and always increase with time. The problem is that in our modern society people often blame these symptoms on their busy schedule and on overwork, when the real fact of the matter is that there is something intrinsically wrong with their body's functioning.

Diabetes

Diabetes is an ailment that we must focus on, because while about equal numbers of men and women suffer from diabetes, women can experience unique symptoms of this disease that men do not. Nearly one tenth of the women in America now suffer from this disease, which makes it a severe health issue for American women. Infection can be a serious problem for women suffering from diabetes, and this includes urinary infections, as well as problems with Candida, or yeast infections. Women who suffer from diabetes also are at far greater risk of experiencing heart issues and problems with the cardio-vascular system. Like all diabetics, a common symptom of the disease is a general inability to heal injuries. However, in women this inability to heal is greater than that experienced by men. Naturally, with the diabetic tendency towards infections, such minor injuries can easily assume far more serious proportions. Circulation of the blood is also affected in diabetic women, especially when they make an attempt to exercise. Any or all of these symptoms are indicators of the disease. However, diabetes is a very serious condition, and diagnosis must always be conducted by a qualified healthcare practitioner.

High blood pressure

High blood pressure in women can be triggered in certain circumstances by hormonal imbalances. Certain research has found that birth control pills have long term effects that can result in high blood pressure. Women have a greater tendency towards high blood pressure after the onset of menopause. Excess weight is dangerous for a woman, because it makes it far more likely that she will develop high blood pressure. Race also seems to be a factor in this ailment, with African American women being far more likely to develop high blood pressure than Caucasians. Controlling high blood pressure can be quite a challenge as many modern drugs to control high blood pressure have been found to have serious side effects, including increasing the risk of diabetes. A more comprehensive approach to controlling this ailment, that takes the entire body into account, seems to be necessary.

Cancer

Cancers that originate in the reproductive system are fairly common in women. For example, more than forty thousand women in America are diagnosed with uterine cancers every year. Cancers of the ovaries are also common, as are cancers of the cervix. The combined numbers of women in America who will be diagnosed with cancers of the breast or reproductive tract are quite staggering. The fact is that healthful lifestyle choices can greatly reduce the risk of contracting many kinds of cancer, but unfortunately people rarely make those choices. Correct nutrition, spirited exercise and avoiding poisonous addictions like smoking and alcohol can massively contribute to preventing cancer. Certain research indicates that reducing environmental stress can also prevent certain kinds of cancer.

Digestive issues

Women also experience more digestive problems, because there is a definite link between these issues and the hormonal cycle in women. The menstrual cycle can affect both digestion and bowel movements, and women who have problems with their digestion around the menstrual cycle can experience these issues consistently for years. While this is perfectly normal, there is much a qualified healthcare practitioner can do to alleviate this issue especially if he works from the point of view of comprehensive healthcare. Medications based on hormones can be especially dangerous to women, because they can trigger exaggerated digestive issues, and many birth control pills fall into this category. And, of course, digestive issues are accentuated during pregnancy because the growing uterus puts pressure upon the entire digestive tract. Women can experience digestive problems during menopause because the hormones are in flux at this stage. As a matter of fact, the hormone replacements prescribed by some doctors can actually make these problems worse. Many digestive issues can be corrected by proper diet combined with a sufficient fluid intake. There are other strategies to further reduce these problems, but they are best undertaken under the supervision of a healthcare practitioner who specializes in a comprehensive discipline of medical care.

Dealing effectively with women's health concerns

Women can become increasingly frustrated as they deal with practitioners of traditional western medicine, because western medicine offers no lasting cure or treatment for the problems we've been enumerating above. Not only does western medicine not seem to understand the unique nature of many women's health issues, but it also has a tendency to focus on treating the symptoms of a condition and to ignore the real, underlying ailment that might be causing those symptoms.[21] Traditional western medicine often ignores the fact that the body is a comprehensive whole, and that an imbalance in one area can have far flung consequences. Focusing on only the symptoms in such circumstances is an extremely short term strategy, and cannot lead to a lasting cure. A discipline like chiropractic is far more effective in treating women's health problems because it has a more comprehensive and more realistic view of healthcare in general and of women's health issues in particular. As explained elsewhere in this chapter, the chiropractic view of health consists of a triangle, in which the three sides support each other. These three sides of the triangle represent the physical or structural aspect of health, the biochemical aspect of health, and the mental/emotional aspect of health. If one side of the triangle is at fault, the other sides of the triangle will also be affected. As an example, extreme stress, which is a mental and emotional issue, can result in cardio-vascular problems. To treat those cardio-vascular problems without treating the stress that is causing them, as a practitioner of traditional western medicine would do, would be

---

[21] New York College of Health Professions. Accessed May 15, 2012. http://www.nycollege.edu/health-care-clinics/our-holistic-approach.php

a mistake. Only a comprehensive discipline like chiropractic, which would treat the cardio-vascular issues while also treating the stresses that underlay them, has any chance of lasting success. The prevalence of women's issues in America today, and the frustration of women who seek treatment from traditional western medicine yet find no lasting cure, make it clear that chiropractic is the need of the hour. Chiropractic's comprehensive approach to health can bring lasting and permanent relief in a host of women's health issues, and a chiropractic physician's attention to crucial aspects of good health such as correct nutrition, exercise and a healthful lifestyle, can guide a woman towards lifelong good health.

Chapter 3:

Pre-Pregnancy Health and Well-Being

You made the decision that it is time to start thinking about getting pregnant. You cannot decide to get pregnant yet, because your body may or may not be in the healthiest condition. When you do make the decision to go forward, you need to commit to getting your body into a natural level of health. This will allow you to potentially conceive sooner, create a better place for your child to develop and even bounce back after pregnancy to a healthy state.

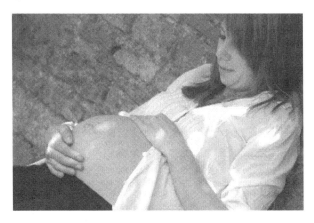

How do you get healthy?

To be healthy, your body needs to balance the three pillars of health. Think of them as a triangle. The triangle cannot stay together unless all three sides are balanced. The same is true for the three elements that create health within the body - the structural, emotional/mental and the chemical makeup of the body. To get healthy, you need to ensure each system of your body is functioning the way it is supposed to. To do that, you need to learn more about the most important components to your body in terms of getting pregnant.

The Endocrine System

You may have thought the most important areas of your body for pregnancy need have to do with your uterus and ovaries. However, it is even more important to focus on the area of your body that will control what happens down there.

According to The Endocrine Society[22], the endocrine system is the body's main system of communicating. It controls as well as coordinates the body's functions. It works along with the nervous system to accomplish this. It also works with your kidneys, liver and pancreas to keep the body functioning. The encocrine system does the following, for example:

- It works to maintain body energy levels
- It helps to respond to the surroundings, including stressors and injuries that occur
- It manages the reproduction system
- It aids in the growth and development of the body

---

[22] Hormone Health Network. Accessed May 15, 2012.
http://www.hormone.org/endo101/.

- It creates an internal balance within the body systems which is called homeostasis

As you can see, the endocrine system plays a very vital role in keeping you healthy. To work, the endocrine system functions through a massive system comprised of glands and organs. They work to produce and then store until the time comes to secrete the various chemicals that flood through the body to tell the body what to do. These chemicals are hormones. They are also chemicals that move into your body's fluids to move to cell groups to create a function. Each type of hormone has a different function within the body.

When the body needs the specifically required hormones, the glands holding these hormones will release them into the bloodstream. The blood carries them to the proper organs, tissues or cells so that the job is done. In order for your body to remain healthy, it must properly maintain the function of the glands so that the proper secretion of hormones can occur.

The problems that can arise are numerous. They often stem from imbalances within the endocrine system. In some cases, the body will release too little or too much of a hormone. In other cases, the glands may not release any. When this happens, it is usually due to an unhealthy balance within the body. Various disorders can cause this to occur.

When a problem with this balance happens, numerous factors can go wrong, including those related to pregnancy. If you want to get pregnant, your body's hormone levels need to be in proper balance to allow for a pregnancy to occur. Many things can happen when the endocrine system is not working properly. This includes problems such as:

- It may take a long time for you to become pregnant.
- Your reproduction system may not work properly and that can result in the inability to conceive or maintain a pregnancy.
- Cell repair drops. This can make it difficult for your body to maintain overall health.
- Regulation of pain is decreased.
- You may lack appetite or, directly the opposite, your metabolism may be not functioning the way it should.

Such issues occur because the nervous system, including the brain, is unable to communicate properly with the rest of the body. The receptors to receive information from hormones cannot function properly. Your organs do not know when to ovulate and they do not know when to allow you to get pregnant. Of course, the endocrine system also plays a role in maintaining every other physiological element of the body.

The Female Endocrine System

When it comes to getting pregnant, the female endocrine system needs to maintain health and balance. It consists of:

- The pituitary gland
- The pineal body
- The thyroid
- The adrenal gland
- The thymus gland
- The pancreas
- The ovaries

Every one of these systems will undergo some level of change during the pregnancy process. These changes are a requirement to allowing the future mother's body to effectively meet all of the needs of the baby during the pregnancy, through the child birthing process and later during breastfeeding.

What's Causing the Problem?

Many women struggle to get pregnant. Many do everything their doctor says and still do not get pregnant regardless of how many times they try to do so. Many things can cause a problem with the endocrine system to lead to complications. Some of these can stop you from getting pregnant whereas others can impact the health of your child once you do. In men, a malfunction of this system can trigger infertility or the inability to maintain a sex drive.

One problem that many women experience is the lack of periods. This is called Amenorrhea. This condition occurs for many reasons but when it is occurring, a woman is unlikely to become pregnant. This can be due to factors such as:

- A low body weight
- Emotional stress
- A low percentage of body fat
- Strenuous exercise that can cause the body to burn through more calories than brought in
- Low calorie intake or fat intake
- Some medical conditions

Other conditions that can prevent a woman from conceiving include infertility, the onset of menopause and hormone related female sexual dysfunction.

The fact is - there is an imbalance in your body's health and as a result, your body cannot function as it should and you cannot get pregnant. Even if you do, this imbalance can affect your unborn child and your health during and after pregnancy. It is critical to get back to a level of health instead.

The Importance of Structural, Chemical and Emotional Health

These three components of health are a must for those who wish to get healthy and to get pregnant. Taking the time and effort to do so will make getting pregnant easier and far more enjoyable. It can even help you avoid many of the complications that women have. Consider the importance of each of these components of health.

Structural Health

The structural health of the body is the physical makeup of the body. The structure of the body is comprised of your joints, muscles, bones and every other physical component. As you can imagine, an injury to your body requires healing and if you do not heal, it can impact your overall health.

When it comes to structural health as it relates to pre-pregnancy, being physically healthy can do many things for your overall well being:

- A healthy body weight can help you to get pregnant.
- The joints of your body need to be strong enough to support the child and additional weight.
- The muscles of your body need to be strong enough to maintain your new body shape and to help encourage your body to get fit after being pregnant.
- Your body's bones need to be strong enough to hold the baby's weight and to adapt properly to cradle the child.

- They can make it easier for you to have a natural pregnancy without a lot of medical intervention necessary.
- A healthy body will make getting pregnant safer and make the environment safer for the unborn child.

Structural health is a must when it comes to maintaining your body's ability to conceive and carry a child. It contributes to your ability to deliver that child, too.

Chemical Health

The chemical composition of the body is a critical component to maintaining your health. It is comprised of any chemical aspect of the body. This includes the hormones racing through your system. It includes the nutritional components of your body. Even the electrical components that trigger how often your heart beats play a role in the chemical makeup of your body. In short, your body does everything through these natural chemical compositions and messages. A malfunction in this area of health can play a big role in pre-pregnancy.

How does chemical health play a role in your ability to get pregnant and to maintain pregnancy?

- The wrong balance of hormones in your body can lead to difficulties getting pregnant. Without the right hormones, it becomes very difficult for this to occur.
- Your body's cells and organs require the proper balance of nutrition. The right nutrients, including vitamins and minerals, are critical to boosting fertility and aiding in a healthy pregnancy.
- The right balance here can also contribute to fewer complications later.

- The right balance of chemicals can contribute to your energy levels.
- Regulation of chemicals such as hormones can create a more even menstrual cycle which encourages conception.
- Low adrenal and thyroid function can also contribute. These can lead to things like post-partum depression, low fertility rate and issues with pregnancy causing premature birth or problems with lactating following pregnancy.

As you can see, there are many aspects that contribute to the chemical aspects of pre-pregnancy. Keep in mind that these chemicals help to regulate every aspect of your body's function, beyond those within the reproductive process.

Emotional/ Mental Health

The third portion of health is the emotional and mental factor. Your emotional health is critical to your well being. If you do not think your mental health plays a role in your ability to get pregnant or to be healthy enough to get pregnant, you may be wrong. Science Daily[23] reports on a study conducted by the Oxford University and US National Institutes of Health. It reports that the biological marker for stress is one reason you may not be getting pregnant. If you are living or working in a stressful environment, your chances of conceiving are significantly fewer than if you were living in a more relaxed environment.

Mental health goes beyond just stress, however. There are many ways that your mental health can be very important to

---

[23] Science Daily. Accessed May 15, 2012.
http://www.sciencedaily.com/releases/2010/08/100817111658.htm.

pre-pregnancy. Consider what the complications can cause, for example:

- Those who suffer from anxiety are often less likely to get pregnant than those who are able to relax.
- Individuals suffering from depression or other types of mental health may have hormonal imbalances that also contribute to the inability to conceive.
- In men, mental and emotional health concerns are likely to contribute to a lower sex drive, erectile dysfunction and infertility.

The fact is, emotional and mental health is just as important as physical and chemical health is. Individuals who do not improve any imbalances or concerns here may find that getting pregnant is very hard to do. It may even contribute to some of the stressors that lead up to pregnancy loss in some women.

What Can Be Done?

When it comes down to it, it can seem nearly frustrating to wonder what can be done to restore health so that your pre-pregnancy body is ready to go. However, it does not have to be overwhelming. It is very possible to balance these three elements of health to help you to achieve your long term health goals. You need to do so in the proper manner, and that is not always the way that most people approach the problem.

Lacking of Traditional Medicine

Traditional medicine is not likely to offer much help to a woman who hopes to get pregnant. In most cases, people do not go to the doctor to discuss their options. They try to get pregnant and most do. There is no medical intervention in most situations.

In these cases, the body is able to adapt to the new fetus as best it can. Though there usually no pre-pregnancy planning, individuals who are healthy enough may experience no problems during the pregnancy. For others, there are complications to consider.

A better approach is to integrate some level of care for individuals prior to getting pregnant. For example, if a woman decides she would like to get pregnant in a year, there should be a period of time in which she is working to restore overall health to her body. Balancing the equation and getting the chemical, structural and emotional elements into place is critical for those who wish to provide the best possible home for their child for the next nine months.

What is lacking in traditional medicine? What could it do better? Here are some considerations to keep in mind.

Obesity

One of the biggest problems facing women today is obesity and being obese or overweight prior to conceiving is a problem.

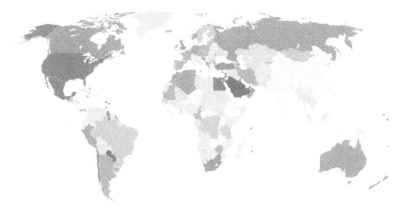

Female obesity statistics – darker areas of the map contain greater concentrations of obese people in the female population

According to Mercola.com[24], one in five pregnant women is obese. This causes high blood pressure and the onset of diabetes in these individuals. Dr. Mercola also notes that there is an increase occurring in the number of pregnancy-related deaths in the United States. For example, he notes that "deaths have tripled in the last 10 years, and overall the maternal mortality rate is 13.3 maternal deaths for every 100,000 births - over four times the US government's 2010 goal of 3.3." These statistics are just from California alone.

Obesity is preventable and treatable. If medical science would encourage or help women to lose weight before conceiving, far fewer deaths would occur. More so, babies would not be born with the health risks they face as a direct result of their mother's weight.

Smoking

Another big no-no that most people are aware of is smoking. However, the body does not need you to stop smoking just when you conceive but in the months leading up to this as well. According to the Oxford Journals[25], a study by the International Journal of Epidemiology notes those women who smoke place an incredibly significant risk on the lives of their children. Those

---

[24] Mercola.com. Accessed May 15, 2012.
http://articles.mercola.com/sites/articles/archive/2010/03/30/there-are-too-many-preventable-deaths-among-new-moms.aspx.
[25] Schlaud, M, and W J. Kleeman. International Journal of Epidemiology. Accessed May 15, 2012.
http://ije.oxfordjournals.org/content/25/5/959.full.pdf.

who do smoke prior to or during pregnancy have a higher risk of their child dying as a result of sudden infant death syndrome.

Other Health Risks

For many women, it is the unknown that is the problem. For those who are struggling to get pregnant, it could be because of current health risks occurring in your body that you do not know about. The following are examples of a lack of traditional medicine providing individuals with the knowledge and treatment they need prior to conceiving:

- Individuals with chemical imbalances, including hormonal imbalances related to ovulation, are likely to struggle to get pregnant. If and when they do, they are at a higher risk for overall health issues during the pregnancy.

- Women, who have structural problems within their body, including those within the reproductive system, are likely to not know about them until they cannot get pregnant. There is no pre-screening for any type of problem in the reproductive system until problems occur.

- Women who suffer from conditions of mental health, including depression, anxiety and other conditions may not be able to conceive or may be at a higher risk for complications related to these factors.

The bottom line is that traditional medicine is often lacking in its ability to provide women with a healthy, balanced body that's ready to conceive and carry a child through the next months without risk.

Are Fertility Treatments Risky?

For many women who cannot conceive, there is no process for learning why. They may have some tests that tell them that they do not have the right balance within the body for pregnancy. In some situations, there are complications that doctors cannot explain. The symptom of the problem is the inability to get pregnant. The solution to it within traditional medicine, on the other hand, is fertility treatments.

There are risks to fertility treatments:

- Some women have a bad reaction to the medications used.

- Others have multiple births which can lead to a greater chance of defects and abnormalities in their children.

- There is a higher risk of ovarian hyper stimulation syndrome occurring.

- Some women experience an emotionally draining ectopic pregnancy and must abort.

- There is a higher risk of birth defects in those who use fertility treatments than those who have a child the natural way.

These reports come from the Human Fertilization and Embryology Authority[26], a division of the UK government.

The problem is not that women are taking these steps to get pregnant. Rather, it is that traditional medicine does nothing to find out what the underlying problem is. What is really causing the woman to be unable to conceive? Though the symptom is obvious, it may be possible to help her to heal and balance health so that she can conceive naturally and therefore reduce the risks to the child and to her overall health.

In traditional medicine, there is a lack of preventative treatment to ensure women are healthy enough to conceive. There is instead a desire to use hormone injections to help women to conceive when their bodies are in less than ideal health. Keeping this in mind, it is fair to say that most women will benefit instead from receiving the proper care and treatment from their doctors before they actually try to conceive.

Though medical science does not provide enough help, there are other ways to ensure you are healthy. With the use of chiropractic care and alternative medicine, women can balance their health and achieve their goals of conceiving healthy children.

Chiropractic and Alternative Care

for Pre-Pregnancy

Turning to a chiropractor for pre-pregnancy care is a good idea. In fact, it is one of the best ways for you to take steps to ensure

[26] Human Fertisilation & Embryology Institute. Accessed May 15, 2012. http://www.hfea.gov.uk/fertility-treatment-risks.html.

your child is coming into a healthy body with every element that he or she needs to maintain health for the next 40 weeks. There are several ways in which chiropractic care and alternative medicine as a whole can help women who are considering becoming pregnant to actually find themselves in that place.

The chiropractic approach is simple - balance the three elements of health and the body will restore natural health necessary for the child's well being and for the mother's as well.

- Chemical health - chiropractic care can help ensure that the body's chemical balance is maintained so that all of the hormones are telling your body what to do properly. Nutrition is managed as well.

- Structural health - this type of care also focuses on ensuring the woman's body is structurally healthy, including the joints, muscles and organs, so that when conception happens, it is ready to support and change to meet the child's needs.

- Emotional health - of course pregnancy does create an emotional toll on most women, but being ready for it by reducing any mental health concerns, can make all of the difference in a woman's health.

The question is, then, how can this be done? There are various ways that a chiropractor can help a woman to be ready for pregnancy.

Traditional Chiropractic Care

One of the ways in which this type of treatment can be highly effective is by balancing the body's health through the nervous system. The nervous system controls every aspect of your body. It starts at the brain and continues through the nerves which travel throughout the body from the spinal column. Messages from your body travel through your nerves to the brain to tell the brain something is wrong. The brain then sends messages to the various organs to respond or do as needed to maintain health.

In some situations, a complication that occurs interferes with this communication highway. When this happens, problems with health occur. This is called a subluxation. It occurs when there is a blockage within the nervous system that keeps the communication from flowing. Chiropractic care can treat this by using a process called an adjustment.

Adjustments do not hurt. They are completely safe to have when a trained chiropractor is using them. By using a small amount of gentle pressure on the areas where subluxation is occurring, it is possible to open up that communication again. This then allows the brain to communicate with that area of the body and to heal naturally.

Doing this prior to getting pregnant can be helpful because it can allow for the body to heal any problems it may have currently.

Additional Alternative Care from Chiropractors

Take it a step further and you will be able to feel great about getting pregnant. Chiropractors also offer a comprehensive set of steps to help ensure your body is ready to conceive. This pre-pregnancy opportunity allows for various alternative care options to be utilized based on your needs to ensure your body is healthy.

Chiropractors will use a variety of tests, for example, to ensure that you are healthy and that if there are any problems they are taken care of long before you conceive. This includes many of the tests medical doctors use such as EKG's, EEG's, diagnostic ultrasounds, blood tests and tests for the lungs. They also use other tests including saliva tests and hair tests that can provide a great deal of information. With this information, the chiropractor can offer suggestions on other types of alternative care that may be beneficial to you:

- Acupuncture - This treatment is highly effective because it works to help with the flow of energy and controlling dependencies. In the hands of a chiropractor it promotes healthy healing and regeneration.

- Nutritional counseling - This is perhaps one of the most important components to any health regimen but it is critical for those who wish to provide their soon-to-be-child with a healthy environment. Chiropractors will use a variety of nutritional counseling options including the use of supplementation to ensure your body is as healthy as it can be.

- Lifestyle Counseling - This is another area that many people can benefit from and do not realize it. With the use of lifestyle counseling, chiropractors can offer advice on how to improve your health, improve your chances of conceiving and ensure that your child has a healthy place to grow and develop.

- Emotional Health - Chiropractors can use a variety of alternative treatments, including NET, Callahan, AK, TBM and other techniques as a way to ensure your emotional health is the best it can be heading into pregnancy. This benefits you as much as the baby.

There is no reason to assume you are healthy enough to conceive. You may look and feel good and you may never have been told by your doctor that there is a problem, but that does not mean your body is in the best possible condition to get pregnant and to maintain a pregnancy for 40 weeks.

Women who seek out preventative care from chiropractic physicians will ensure their body's have a balance of health present. This is a critical step in ensuring you are doing all you can to provide your child with a healthy environment to grow. However, it is also beneficial to the mother. With the proper treatment prior to getting pregnant, you are less likely to experience complications as well as limitations during those months. Afterwards, your body is better able to bounce back and provide for the needs of the child. Chiropractic care can be one of the best solutions for those women who want a healthy pregnancy.

Chapter 4:

Pregnancy

Pregnancy is an exciting and exhilarating time of life. Both men and women can share in this joy, but once the reality settles in, it is the woman who needs to ensure her body and baby remain healthy for the next 40 weeks. Pregnancy is a great time to take a look at your overall health and to determine if you are doing everything you can to keep your child healthy.

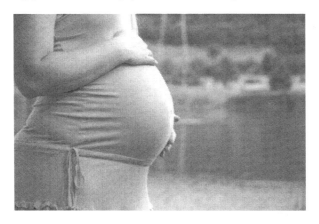

Many mothers-to-be would do anything to ensure that their child is born with ten fingers and ten toes, and with everything in between being just fine. However, many do not realize there are steps they can take to ensure this happens, or at least to give the child the best possible ability to avoid complications. It is also important to consider the mother's needs. Though a lot of the focus during pregnancy is on the baby, the mother's body is one of the most vital aspects of maintaining that child's health. Therefore, the mother's health also needs to be maintained properly in order for everything to go just right.

In the best of situations, mothers-to-be have gone through a pre-pregnancy clearance and stage in which they have done whatever they can to ensure the health and well being of their body so that pregnancy itself goes well. If not, it is still possible to remain healthy and even to improve health during this time to encourage development and maintain health for both the baby and the mother. The key to achieving this is to know what is happening within the body and then to use every possible resource available to ensure any problems are dealt with in an effective manner. For women, there is no doubt that pregnancy is a trying time, but when you take steps to get healthy you can see it as an opportunity to do something grand for the world.

The actual stages of pregnancy change a woman's body significantly. There are aspects to pregnancy that require the body to work as it was designed to in order to create a healthy place for the child. In order for your body to meet these demands, you need to understand the vast number of changes that will occur once you get pregnant. Numerous systems of your body will be taxed and pushed to the limit. And, in some cases, you may find yourself overwhelmed with the process.

There is something you can do about this, though. With the aid of a chiropractic physician, you will be able to strengthen your body and mind to ensure that you can give your child everything it needs. In addition, you should know what steps to take beyond what medical science in the United States says you to ensure your baby and your body remains healthy. Even if you do everything your medical doctor says, you may not be doing enough. That's why you need additional advice and guidance from chiropractic physicians who focus on giving the body back its natural ability to heal itself and its natural ability to reproduce.

Structural Changes During Pregnancy

Most women understand that there will be changes to a body as a direct result of getting pregnant. The most obvious is the growing child within her. However, there is more to it than just that.

The structure of the body is the physical components that make it up, including the bones, muscles and every system in between. The changes that occur with your structural system are dependent on many factors, including the previous condition of the body, the location of the baby, your weight, your height and many other elements.

These structural changes need to happen because they need to make room for your growing child. The changes bring with them stress on virtually all aspects of your body, especially the muscles, bones and joints. Your spine and pelvis are likely to bare the most of it, but in some cases painful complications can occur throughout the body.

Take a look at what happens during pregnancy to the body as things change. In general, many women suffer from the following complications that come from these changes in the structure of the body:

- The lower back begins to curve. This is painful and it can be debilitating. It occurs because of the shifting of the bones and muscles to make room for the baby within the pelvic region, but any movement of the spine further than its normal range of motion can be very taxing.

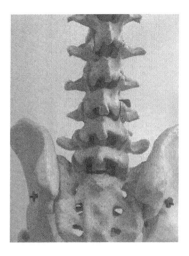

The bones of the lower spine

- In some situations, the bones and joints do not move as they should, which can cause problems not just during the pregnancy but also later during delivery. For example, if the pelvis does not open properly during delivery, this can cause long-term damage and lead to significant pain. This can happen for many reasons including simply misalignments within the body.
- As these changes occur, the body's nervous system can get in the way. For example, as the joints, ligaments and muscles move and flex to make room, they can cause an impediment of the flow of information from the nerves to the brain. When this happens, you may end up

dealing with complications including irritation and pain. In other cases, the organs and glands do not function as they should. If a person's body is already out of alignment heading into pregnancy, this can worsen this condition.

There are many instances in which something can go wrong. Though it is not possible to stop or prevent everything from occurring, giving your body a healthy, functioning structure, can reduce some of the complications during and after pregnancy. According to the National Institutes of Health[27], the following are the most common health complications that can complicate a pregnancy:

- Heart disease
- High blood pressure
- Autoimmune disorders
- Kidney problems
- Cancers
- Infections
- Diabetes
- Sexually transmitted diseases

In addition, some people will suffer from conditions such as gestational diabetes and Rh incompatibility during pregnancy. Many women also deal with back pain, fatigue, nausea and emotional stress during pregnancy. The body's change and

---

[27] Medline Plus. Accessed May 17, 2012.
http://www.nlm.nih.gov/medlineplus/healthproblemsinpregnancy.html.

sometimes its inability to change in the right way can trigger these types of health complications and risks.

How are you going to provide a safe pregnancy? To do so, you need to ensure your body is healthy, structurally, to ensure any conditions you may have or any conditions you could develop are controllable.

The structural health of the body can reduce the risk of many complications. The bones, joints, ligaments and muscles can work properly and help ensure the pregnancy goes the way it should without risks.

Chemical Changes During Pregnancy

Perhaps even larger than the structural changes during pregnancy are the chemical ones. These are the situations in which the body's chemical makeup - including the hormones produced by the body and the support of nutrition in the body.

Chemicals make up the function of the body. They tell the body what to do, as directed by the secretion of hormones. Consider the body's makeup. It is made up of cells which require nutrition to do their job. Nutrition, including vitamins and minerals, provides a very important resource for cells. To perform specific tasks, these cells require specific types of nutrients.

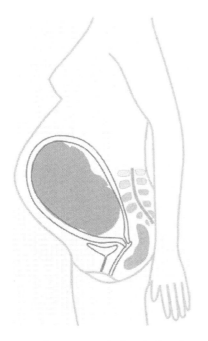

Pregnancy brings complex structural, chemical and mental emotional changes to a woman's body

When a woman gets pregnant, the needs of the body are intensified. There are some types of nutrients she needs more during pregnancy than she did prior to getting pregnant. At the same time, she also needs to consume more calories in order to provide the body with energy to help encourage the child to grow and to feed the child's cells.

Nutritional Needs During Pregnancy

The nutritional needs of a woman during pregnancy are very important. Without these needs being met, the end result could be a lack of overall health and well being for the child. The following are the suggestions in the nutrients women need during pregnancy, as well as later when they are breastfeeding, to maintain health, from a study done by The Ohio State University:[28]

- Protein is an important component for building the muscles to hold the baby, the breasts to feed the baby, the uterus to protect the child and the blood supply. It also is necessary for the development of the child. The recommendations for women are about 71 grams per day.
- Folate is an important vitamin for women because it helps to build protein tissues. Low levels are linked to numerous health complications in children including conditions such as spina bifida. Women need about 600 micrograms each day during pregnancy.
- Calcium is also critical to help build the mother's bones and to help the bone development in the child as well. Pregnant women need 1000 milligrams each day if they are over the age of 19.
- A low level of iron can cause numerous defects in children. It is necessary for the development of healthy blood supplies in the body. Pregnant women almost always need supplementation to reach the requirement of 27 milligrams daily.
- Zinc levels need to be maintained as well. Low numbers create a higher risk of having a child with health complications. 11 milligrams per day is the recommended dose for pregnant women.

---

[28] The Ohio State University. Accessed May 17, 2012. http://ohioline.osu.edu/hyg-fact/5000/pdf/5573.pdf.

In addition to this, women also need to do the following to ensure they are getting enough of the nutrients their body needs:

- Eat a variety of foods from a range of food groups.
- Ensure they are getting enough calories for adequate weight gain in the child.
- Get at least 30 grams of dietary fiber in their diet daily
- Drink enough water to ensure the cells are fully hydrated, at least eight glasses per day
- No use of alcohol or tobacco

The problem is most pregnant women do not get this level of healthy nutrients. The American diet is a high calorie diet that offers very little nutrition to most pregnant mothers. Medical doctors state that taking a prenatal vitamin is enough to provide the nutrition that is missed, but that is not the case. In short, women who want to have healthy children need to balance the chemical health of their bodies to achieve it. To do that, they need to consider nutrition a very important component to their overall health and well being. Proper chemical balance can lead to a healthy body that reacts the way it needs to for the child's well being.

There is another side of chemical health that is just as important, though. It is also important to manage the needs of your endocrine system.

The Endocrine System

The endocrine system is a large, complex network that controls many of the functions of the body. When working properly, the endocrine system tells the body exactly what it needs to do to be ready to care for this child. Here's how it works, according to Clermont College:[29]

The body's nervous system, which includes the nerves and the brain, sends an electrical message to the various portions of the body to control functions there. The endocrine system has a similar job but instead of using electrical impulses, it uses chemicals to communicate. These chemicals are manufactured by the body and are known as hormones. Hormones are synthesized for a specific reason and when they enter the body, they tell the organs to perform in a specific way. The endocrine gland is the gland that controls this production of hormones, which then enter into the bloodstream and travel to the locations where the appropriate organs are.

During pregnancy, the endocrine system needs to change enough to support he needs of the child and the mother. It is stressed. In most cases, it can work properly to ensure that every organ in the body is doing what it needs to in order to provide the pregnancy with the necessary support.

Here are some of the changes that occur in the endocrine system during pregnancy. It is clear just how important it is for the body to maintain healthy endocrine function when you can see just how many ways it can affect the pregnancy:

- The parathyroid gland - This gland will increase in size slightly during pregnancy. It is also vitally important to pregnancy because it helps meet the needs of calcium in the baby. This increase in calcium requirement is necessary for healthy development.

---

[29] Clermont College. Accessed May 17, 2012.
http://biology.clc.uc.edu/courses/bio105/endocrin.htm.

- The posterior pituitary gland - Closer to the end of the pregnancy, this gland kicks into gear. At this time, it begins to secrete a hormone called oxytocin. This hormone is produced in the hypothalamus which then tells the posterior pituitary gland to start working. When the appropriate time comes, this gland will kick in to initiate labor.

- The anterior pituitary gland - When birth occurs, this gland goes to work. It secretes a hormone called prolactin. When this enters the body, it helps to stimulate the production of breast milk so the mother can begin to nurse her child nearly right away.

- The adrenal gland - It does not change in size during pregnancy but it does increase the production of cortisol, which is helpful in times of stressful situations, both long term and short term. In terms of the effect on the pregnancy, it helps to maintain sugar in the plasma, repairs tissues, manufactures enzymes, works as an anti-inflammatory, helps with allergic actions and helps to break down glucose.

Perhaps the most unique change to the body with regard to the endocrine system and hormones is the placenta itself. It works as a temporary, separate endocrine gland during pregnancy. It will continue to work throughout pregnancy to create the necessary changes in the body. At about ten to twelve weeks into a pregnancy, it begins to produce a large amount of estrogen and progesterone. In addition, the placenta works to ensure the fetus continues to grow to a healthy level. It helps to control the activity of the uterus as well. In fact, the placenta is one of the most important working glands within the body during the entire maternal change.

Effective management of the body's endocrine system is critical in maintaining the pregnancy and maintaining overall health. If a woman's endocrine system is not functioning as it should, this can cause a number of different problems throughout the pregnancy and even affect the well being of the child. The chemical balance within the body is critical to maintain for these reasons.

The chemical health of the body is dependent on nutrition and a highly functional endocrine system, yet many women have no idea what they need to do to maintain or build on health. This can leave them with higher risks than are necessary.

Medical Care Isn't There

Everyone knows that a woman needs to see the doctor and have prenatal care when it comes to pregnancy. The fact is, this type of care needs to start long before a woman actually gets pregnant. However, that is often not what occurs.

According to the Health Resources and Services Administration's Maternal and Child Health Bureau[30], international infant mortality rates are not the lowest in the United States. In fact, in 2000, the US ranked 27th among industrialized nations in terms of the number of live births and infant deaths that occur annually.

In a country where medical treatment is available and there are numerous programs for prenatal care, this seems like a shockingly high number.

---

[30] Child Health USA 2004. Accessed May 17, 2012.
http://www.mchb.hrsa.gov/mchirc/chusa_04/pages/0405iimr.htm.

Here are some additional statistics from the US Department of Health and Human Services that may be worrisome to many people:[31]

- One million American women have babies each year in the United States without getting adequate medical attention.

- Babies who are born to mothers who received no prenatal care in that pregnancy were three times more likely to have a low birth weight.

- Babies who were born to mothers who received no prenatal care in pregnancy are also five times more likely to die than those whose mothers did receive the appropriate level of care.

There are many programs available for women to get help, but even when they do, they may not be getting enough. Medical doctors screen for basic hormone levels and overall health. Physicals that look at the overall health of the structural body of the woman are very rarely considered even though this can contribute to a lack of well being for both the mother and the child. Even further, many women have no idea if they are at risk for any type of complication because their medical doctors do not tell them.

If there is a problem found, another issue is symptoms being treated but not the underlying cause. This leaves many women struggling to balance medications and bed rest when they are

---

[31] HRSA. Accessed May 17, 2012.
http://www.mchb.hrsa.gov/programs/womeninfants/prenatal.html.

unable to fully cope with the situation. This limitation is one that many women are simply struggling with and have no idea why.

The lacking of appropriate medical treatment in the US for pregnancy is worrisome. With millions of children born each year, it is imperative that women have healthy bodies prior to the pregnancy, maintain this through the pregnancy and have appropriate treatment for their needs to avoid complications. It may not be possible to obtain this type of help from a traditional doctor but there are other solutions that can help you to overcome these risks.

Chiropractic and Alternative Treatments for Pregnancy

Pregnancy is an exciting time but it is also time to consider your overall goals for your child. You want a healthy body and you want your child to have every opportunity to be healthy. This is why it is critical to take the steps necessary to get healthy right now. Chiropractic care can do that for you. Many chiropractic physicians provide services to those who are pregnant because the need is greater now than in other situations.

What Can Chiropractic Care Offer?

Chiropractic care is a form of care that involves treating the whole body. The goal is not to focus just on treating a person's symptoms as with traditional medicine. Rather, it has a goal of balancing the three main components of health to offer an overall level of wellness that allows the body to use its natural ability to heal to overcome any limitations.

There are three areas in which focus is needed in order for a pregnant woman to really be healthy and to give the body its natural ability to heal from any limitations:

- Structural Health - This focuses on the overall needs for a woman's body and ensuring the joints, bones and muscles are all working in the proper way. The structural health of a women's body, as mentioned earlier, is critical to supporting a growing child and helping her to maintain her health and wellness long term.

- Chemical Health - Also as discussed earlier, the chemical health of a woman's body is critical when it comes to achieving long term health and wellness. Without a proper balance of the chemicals in her body, it will be hard it to respond to the needs of the baby or to the woman.

- Emotional Health - Mental or emotional health is just as vitally important to well being. The emotional health of a woman during pregnancy can change as the chemicals racing through her body change. In addition, this is a trying time that can be filled with times of depression and anxiety. Emotional health balance is critical to maintaining a successful pregnancy.

In order for a person to be healthy, all three of these areas need to be balanced. If one is not balanced, then the risks of developing problems are larger. The question is, how can you balance them? That's done by chiropractic physicians.

How Chiropractic Can Help

Chiropractic physicians can offer numerous types of treatments to enable a person to improve health and to balance the three areas listed above. One of the most common methods is to address any types of structural concerns using adjustments. Adjustments are treatments in which the chiropractor will use a gentle amount of pressure on specific areas of the body. This is done because of something called subluxation.

Subluxation occurs when a problem occurs between the pathways of information that pass through the nervous system. The brain sends messages through the nerves which run through the spinal column to the various areas of the body. This allows for messages to easily travel from the brain to the muscles or organs so they can take action. However, in some cases, structural problems can occur in which something blocks this passageway. Problems can occur that can lead to a lack of communication within the nervous system. When this happens, subluxation occurs. That is the point of the problem.

By using adjustments in the right locations, it is possible to overcome these areas of subluxation. When that is done, the brain is then again able to communicate properly with the body because this pathway is opened. During pregnancy, it is quite common for subluxations to occur because of the numerous changes happening within the structure of the body.

Additional Ways Chiropractors Aid During Pregnancy

As mentioned, it is critical to balance all components of health during pregnancy. For that reason, chiropractic physicians often offer more help than just fixing the structural concerns of the body. One of the first steps for the chiropractor will be to better understand what is happening within the body and where any areas of concern are occurring. Chiropractors have a large number of tests and processes they can use to determine if there are any problems occurring.

The use of tests such as CAT scans, x-rays, MRIs, diagnostic ultrasounds and blood tests are all similar to those that medical doctors do, though chiropractic physicians are usually looking for more information. In addition, chiropractors often do other tests including tests such as saliva testing and hair testing to better understand what is occurring within the body.

Once there is an understanding, the chiropractic physician will offer the proper types of alternative treatments that can benefit the individual. Some of those treatments include the following.

- Acupuncture may be an option for some women. It can help in the process of regeneration as well as healthy healing. It can also help to open up energy channels.

- Lifestyle counseling is another important tool that chiropractors can use to help pregnant women and it is one of the most important. By addressing any areas in which the woman is struggling that are negatively impacting their health it is possible to provide a healthier outcome during the pregnancy.

- Supplementation is one of the most critical components of ensuring a child is healthy throughout the pregnancy and that the woman's needs are being met. This includes using non-synthetic supplementation that is better to the child than the prenatal vitamins a medical doctor may provide as treatment for nutritional needs.

When it comes to ensuring a child is developing properly and that the mother is able to be as healthy as possible throughout pregnancy, it is necessary to build whole health - something which cannot take place unless all three areas of health are at their highest levels. To ensure this happens, women who are pregnant need to seek out the services of a chiropractic physician who can offer structural, chemical and emotional treatments to meet the demands of the woman and the child during pregnancy. It is safe and it is one of the best steps a woman can take to ensure a pregnancy goes the way she wants it to go and that the best possible outcome takes place.

Chapter 5:

Post Pregnancy

A woman's body has one of the most important jobs in helping to create life. Yet, pregnancy is not a simple process and it does have an incredible impact on a person's overall health and well being. After giving birth, even the healthiest person going into the pregnancy will now find complications to deal with. There's a baby to take care of and that puts even more demands on the mother's body.

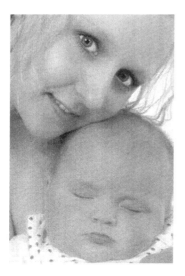

Women need to take a step back after giving birth to ensure they have what it takes to continue to help the child grow and to develop through breastfeeding but also because they need to allow their own body to start the healing process. Getting back into shape is not just a physical step. It entails doing much more for the body as a whole. To do this, many women exercise or they restrict their diets at a time when they simply need improved nutrition or to allow her body time to overcome the massive changes it went through.

After having a child, virtually every system of the body is in a state of change. It is up to the woman to take steps to improve overall health to get over these changes.

- Menstruation may be heavier or it may change compare to before the pregnancy. It can be taxing during those first few months.
- Your endocrine system is adjusting to the different demands of the body now that the child is born. Your hormone levels may be all over the place until things get back into control.
- There is now a new demand of the body to produce milk for the child. Lactation is a critical step in post pregnancy and it is no small feat either.
- Your body has to heal from the strange positions the bones and joints where in while carrying extra weight. Your body needs to strengthen.
- Your mental health is changing too. Now, you are not the center of attention but the demands on you to feel perfect are increasing.

There is a lot to think about and to go through, but when you put together a healthy treatment plan to get you back to where you want and need to be, you may find that everything is easier to manage. Many women need to seek out medical care and support after pregnancy but many do not do so.

It is first important to understand what is occurring within your body and what the new demands of it are. It is also important to realize the amount of work your body is undertaking right now so you can improve your chances of healing and getting back into shape. Then, you need the tools appropriate to make this all happen. As you will see, it is not the medical doctor you should be striving to see and get help from but rather from chiropractic care and alternative treatments available through chiropractors. These can be the best tools available to you if you want to improve your overall health.

Breastfeeding and Lactation

One of the biggest demands on the body after pregnancy is breastfeeding. Lactation begins to occur nearly right away after a woman gives birth. The endocrine system sends out a message to tell the proper glands to secrete the appropriate hormone to get the lactation process underway. It does this naturally and without any encouragement from you. However, lactation is a demanding process on the body.

The Importance of Breastfeeding

Though demanding on a woman's body, breastfeeding is one of the most important nutrition resources for the child. It is recommended that babies feed exclusively on breast milk for the first six months of life. The US Department of Health and Human Services Office on Women's Health[32] notes the following

---

[32] Womens Health. Accessed May 18, 2012.
http://www.womenshealth.gov/breastfeeding/.

about a child's need for breast milk: "Early breast milk is liquid gold - Known as liquid gold, colostrum, is the thick yellow first breast milk that you make during pregnancy and just after birth. This milk is very rich in nutrients and antibodies to protect your baby." Other benefits of breast milk include:

- Being the perfect type of nutrition for the child, it has the perfect amount of fat, sugar, water and protein a child needs.
- It is easier to digest for the baby than any other form.
- It helps to fight diseases because of the presence of the mother's hormones, cells and antibodies. Formula-fed babies are more likely to develop lower respiratory infections, obesity, asthma, type 2 diabetes and necrotizing.
- Mother's benefit too from the ability to lose weight faster, remaining healthier from the improved diet and in saving money.

As incredibly important as breastfeeding is, the problem is that not enough children receive it. The Centers for Disease Control released its annual Breast Feeding Report Card for 2011. It showed that only 14.8 percent of babies are exclusively breast fed for six months and that only 35 percent are exclusively breast feeding at three months of age.[33]

Why is this happening? Why are there not more women taking the necessary steps to care for their child? It could be that only 5 percent of US infants are born in hospitals that are Baby

---

[33] Center for Disease Control. Accessed May 18, 2012.
http://www.cdc.gov/breastfeeding/pdf/2011BreastfeedingReportCard.pdf.

Friendly, according to the same report. Those hospitals are those that take extensive steps to encourage breastfeeding. This means that more children than ever start off without the proper nutrition for their bodies when there is nearly always a perfect source available to them.

There are many benefits to breastfeeding. The National Institute of Child Health and Human Development[34] offer the following benefits to breastfeeding:

- These children have fewer deaths during the first year and fewer illnesses than children who are fed formula.
- Some nutrients protect against childhood illnesses and infections including middle ear infections, lung infections and diarrhea.
- Breastfeeding has been show to improve a child's cognitive skills.

Lactation's Demands

While keeping this in mind is important, it is also critical to understand what happens with lactation and how it changes the demands of the body in women after pregnancy. Consider what happens and changes when women breastfeed.

After birth, lactation occurs in a woman's breasts. This is the secretion of a type of milk from the mammary glands. In the 24th week of pregnancy and onwards, the body produces hormones that help to stimulate the woman's milk duct system which is found within her breasts. The following hormones play a role in this process:

---

[34] NIHCD. Accessed May 18, 2012.
http://www.nichd.nih.gov/health/topics/Breastfeeding.cfm.

- Progesterone encourages the growth of the alveoli and lobes. At the time of birth, these levels drop to encourage the production of milk.
- Estrogen stimulates the milk ducts and, as with progesterone, the levels drop just before birth to encourage production of milk.
- Prolactin is another hormone and this one also causes changes in the milk ducts. In addition, it helps to increase insulin resistance and balance.

Numerous other hormones contribute to the process. All of this is in the goal of helping to prepare the breasts to deliver milk to a child. By the sixth month of pregnancy, the woman's breasts are ready to produce milk. Lactation will begin at the onset of birth.

Once this begins to occur, stimulation to the breasts causes a rise in prolactin levels. They peak for about 45 minutes and then return to their normal level. This helps the alveoli in the breasts to make milk. Along with the milk the child receives, it also gets the antibodies and natural protections that the mother already has. This provides health benefits as well as overall protection from the onset of infections and viruses present in the world itself.

Lactation is a big process and one that will be called upon hundreds of times in the next few months. As a result, a woman's body needs to be ready to provide the child with everything it needs. This is especially true as the chemical composition of breast milk is constantly changing to meet the needs and demands of the child.

There are complications that can occur, however. Sometimes, problems with regulation of hormones can limit the amount of milk produced. Some women will produce too much while others will produce too little. In addition, without the necessary calories and nutrition in the woman's diet, the child's milk may not be as nutritious as it would be otherwise. Just as the child fed on the same caloric and nutrition ingestion that the mother took in during pregnancy, the same occurs in breastfeeding. If a mother is not eating a healthy diet that offers the proper levels of nutrients to the child, the child's system is unable to benefit as well as it could be.

This is why breastfeeding as a healthy woman is critical. If there are any structural concerns with the milk ducts or the glands in the body, the child will not receive the best source of nutrients for it. At the same time, if the child is not given the opportunity to nurse he or she is missing out on the one source of nutrients on the planet that is best for its health and development.

As mothers, most women want to give their child everything they need, but they may not know the value of breastfeeding or believe they can do it. However, breastfeeding after pregnancy is a critical step to encourage the well being of a child.

Restoring Health After Pregnancy

There is a great deal of thought and planning in helping a new child to be healthy but not enough attention is put on helping the mother to be healthy as well. After pregnancy, her body is very different than what it was prior to pregnancy. Through proper treatment, it is possible to restore health and to improve overall well being. However, many woman have no idea the amount of change occurring.

Take a look at the three components that make up health and how they change during pregnancy. After pregnancy, it is important to restore health to these areas in order to encourage well being and development in the mother.

Structural Changes

There are significant changes to a woman's body after pregnancy. During pregnancy, the body changes shape, with bones, joints and muscles changing and moving to allow for support of the child.

- The structure of the body needs to improve to ensure proper health and structural support for the mother. It needs to shift back to the place it was before.
- Epidurals are a common type of pain relieving medication given to women through the spinal column during labor. However, they can leave their mark on a woman's body causing pain and discomfort for years to come.
- Antibiotics are often given to help prevent illness from infection during birth but they can also cause problems within the body.
- C-sections, when necessary, create large cuts in the abdominal wall to allow for the child to be delivered through this opening. Not only does it need to heal, but the body's strength and structural support is at risk.

All of these structural changes to a woman's body need to be improved upon in order to allow her to heal and gain back the strength and support necessary. For example, if nothing is done to improve the problems caused by an epidural pain and discomfort can continue long term. This can also interfere with the nervous system's function not just in the back region but throughout a woman's entire body.

The structural changes during pregnancy can be hard to see and understand but they do have a significant impact on the well being of the woman right after birth and in the months and years later. Proper restorative treatment is critical.

Chemical Changes

The body also changes through pregnancy in terms of the chemical balance. After pregnancy, there are still chemicals in the body that are changing the way it functions. Proper balance is necessary to restore the health and well being of the individual.

One component of the chemical changes that are required during the period of time after pregnancy has to do with the calorie and nutritional changes that are different for women after having a child. For lactation to occur, the body needs to receive the appropriate nutrients. This includes the following:

- At least 1800 calories per day is necessary. Women who lose more than one to four pounds while breastfeeding may not be getting enough calories.

- Calcium needs are just as high after pregnancy as they are during. Women need to eat calcium rich foods throughout the day, usually four to five servings.

- Protein is also in demand. Lean protein is a must throughout breastfeeding. Aim to include at least two servings daily of a high source of protein.

Aside from this, nutritional balance may require additional help through supplementation. This is depending on the individual's needs.

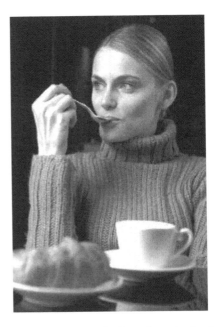

Aside from these elements of the chemical change, keep in mind that the body's hormone levels need to regulate. While it is necessary for lactation to continue, it will also be important for a woman's body to get back to health by properly balancing hormones within the body.

Emotional Changes

One of the least talked about but most important changes occurring in a woman's body after delivering a baby are the emotional or mental changes. The Mayo Clinic[35] reports that the causes of post partum depression, one of the biggest risks for women who have just given birth, include the following:

- The physical changes within the body including the significant drop of hormones estrogen and progesterone, which leads to a feeling of being tired and depressed

- Demands of the child including those of other siblings, as well as the taxing on the body as a result of breast feeding,

- The requirements of financial bills, lack of support and overall frustrations with new lifestyle changes

- Emotional factors including those stemming from being sleep deprived and simply overwhelmed can cause emotional instability

It is clear that many women suffer from emotional concerns after pregnancy and it may seem as though they come from every direction. However, without the appropriate help for the mother, these problems can lead to long term complications for women including severe depression and anxiety.

Women need to put focus on healing their bodies fully after having a baby. However, there is almost no attention given to the mother's needs after a child is born. In fact, the first thing

---

[35] Mayo Clinic. Accessed May 18, 2012.
http://www.mayoclinic.com/health/postpartum-depression/DS00546/DSECTION=causes.

women schedule after having a child is the well checkups for the child. Most do not even see their own doctor for months. This can lead to complications in every area of a person's health including the structural, chemical and the emotional makeup of these people. That can lead to problems that follow women throughout life.

Back Pain

This may be a result of the delivery of the baby. It may also be enhanced or a continuation of something that occurred before or during pregnancy. Be aware of all that is going on with your body and especially your back during this time.

Why Is It Happening?

Why do so many women never get the level of care they need after having a child? Why do so many children suffer because they were not given breast milk when it is so clearly a beneficial source of nutrients and poses little to no risk or limitation to the mother? These concerns can be traced by to a lacking within the American medical industry. In short, there is little to no help available to women and there is even less education on these subjects.

It is widely known that in third world countries, young children are often breastfed exclusively for their first few months. The reason for this may be simple - it is a free source of nutrition for the child. However, in many industrialized, modern cultures, breastfeeding is no longer seen as a culturally acceptable option. The thought of seeing a mother breastfeed is something that outrages many people. It seems indecent and, even when breast pumps are in use many women see the entire process as far too inconvenient.

It is far easier to use formula to feed a child. Many of these formulas even promise the public that they are just like mother's milk or contain the same nutrients found in mother's milk. The problem here is that this is just not accurate. While these formulas may contain a high amount of nutrients, they still do not contain the other chemicals and antibodies that are so vitally important to the child. That is why many of them are sorely lacking.

Considering why women face so many obstacles in overcoming the structural, chemical and emotional challenges after giving birth, the lack of available medical care is a big problem. Many women do not have the ability to go back to the medical doctor right after giving birth because they:

- Are not told or educated about the needs of their body after this point

- Are not encouraged to do so by insurance companies which will pay for follow up care at six weeks only

- Do not have easily accessible options

- Only go to the doctor when there is a problem that needs attention

Then, when there is a problem and the woman does go to the doctor, the problem is rarely solved. Rather, medical doctors often do not know there is a problem and when there is, they treat the symptoms rather than solving the underlying cause of the concern. This is a big problem for women who need help physically to get fit after having a child.

While this is a big problem and for many women, there does not seem like there is anything that can be done. However, with the aid of chiropractic physicians, there is something that can be done to change the health and well being of women after giving birth to solve any health problems that exist within the body.

Chiropractic and Alternative Treatments

Medical doctors may not provide enough treatment for the underlying cause of the health problems many women have after pregnancy, but chiropractic physicians do. In fact, you should visit a chiropractor for care prior to getting pregnant, through pregnancy and after. That's because these professionals focus on improving health by balancing those three elements discussed earlier.

When the body's structural, chemical and emotional needs are being met after pregnancy, the body is better able to achieve its overall health goals. In short, your body has the natural ability to heal and overcome the changes and demands of pregnancy, breast feeding any other challenges if it is given the proper abilities to do so. In order to accomplish this, you need to focus on the following solutions.

- The structural needs of the body, including the muscles, bones and joints, require attention after pregnancy. This is done through subluxation treatment, discussed below. By ensuring that the body has the ability to communicate properly and to heal any structural changes or injuries is critical to overall health.

- The chemical needs of the body are just as important. These include the nutritional needs of the body as well as the regulation of hormones. Women need to have the appropriate treatments to ensure these chemical balances are in line.

- The emotional or mental health of a woman is just as important. This focuses on the mental health of a woman such as anxiety and depression. These are both big factors in helping women to be able to manage the demands of post pregnancy life.

There is one thing to remember about these three elements. They cannot be maintained individually. In other words, you cannot be emotional healthy if your hormones are not inline. You cannot be structural fit if your chemical needs are not being met. In short, the three elements, when aligned and balanced, will allow the body to appropriately communicate and handle the demands of post pregnancy with ease.

That's because the body has a natural ability to heal. When these three elements are together, balanced and focused, then it is possible to overcome any of the changes and trauma the body must deal with after having a child.

In order for you to get to this point, though, there needs to be a focus on obtaining the appropriate health treatment. This is done through chiropractic care and through alternative treatments. Chiropractic physicians can help you to achieve these goals.

Subluxation and Adjustments

In order to improve the structural health of the body, it may be necessary to locate areas of subluxation and to take steps to improve them. Subluxation is a type of blockage. To understand how it happens, consider how the nervous system works.

The nervous system consists of the brain as well as a massive passageway of nerves. When the brain wants an action to take place in an organ or muscle, it will send an electrical impulse down the appropriate nerve through the spinal column and to the area where the action needs to occur. The nerves can also send messages back to the brain when there is a problem so that the appropriate improvement can occur.

When there is some type of blockage that occurs and interferes with this communication, this is called a subluxation. This is why things like epidurals or c-sections can lead to long term problems for individuals. If there is some break in the communication process, chiropractors can help by performing an adjustment. Adjustments are the use of gentle pressure on the appropriate areas to get the flow of communication back to the level it was at so that structural improvements can occur.

Alternative Treatments Available from Chiropractic Physicians

It is further possible to make improvements to the body's health by using alternative medicines aside from subluxation treatment. Chiropractors can use numerous types of alternative medicines and treatments to help make improvements.

First, to find out what the current health of the body is, the chiropractor is likely to run a series of tests to better understand where any problems are occurring. By using tests such as EKG's, CAT scans, blood tests and many other procedures that medical doctors also use, the chiropractor can gain more information about what is really happening within the body. These tests help to chiropractor to learn about the symptoms of any problems you may be happening.

What sets apartment medical science from these types of alternative treatments and chiropractic care is that the chiropractic physician goes further. He or she does not treat just the symptoms but instead looks for the underlying problem to solve it. This may be done in numerous ways. Here are some examples.

- With the use of acupuncture, chiropractors can help to improve energy flow as well as promote healthy healing. This process can also help in tissue regeneration.

- Often times, lifestyle choices in woman after pregnancy can contribute to the health concerns they have. For example, problems with smoking or being overweight can be big factors in dealing with health maintenance. With the aid of a chiropractic physician, lifestyle coaching is available to make significant improvements in these underlying problems.

- Perhaps one of the biggest improvements that chiropractors can offer for chemical and emotional well being is to adjust a person's diet. Through improving nutritional health, if this is a problem, many breastfeeding mothers will get healthy again. It is often necessary for chiropractic physicians to use non-synthetic forms of supplementation to help in these needs.

As you can see, taking care of your body post pregnancy is one of the most important things women can do for themselves as well as for their child. However, modern medical science does not provide enough attention to the underlying problems occurring to cause limitations and chronic conditions. Women who experience pain, discomfort, depression, anxiety or the inability to lactate needs help from chiropractors to determine what the underlying cause of the problem is.

With this help, they can then count on receiving the necessary treatments to get back to balancing those three elements that are necessary. By balancing structural, chemical and emotional needs of women after having a baby, women can restore overall health by allowing the body to use its natural ability to heal.

Chapter 6:

Common Developmental Issues in Childhood and the Role of Chiropractic Care

Children have unique needs. They follow a developmental pattern that is starkly different from that of adults. Five to six centuries ago, children were regarded only as a miniature version of an adult.

Portraits and pictures by famous artists in the Western tradition clearly depicted children as having the same physical structure as an adult, but just scaled down. The fallacy of this idea was slow to be recognized.

However, paintings of the renaissance era began to show children as having distinctly different characteristics. The bigger heads, longer trunk and short limbs began to appear in the paintings.

The fetus develops in some particular sequence in the womb and the process of development continues after birth. The skeletal and the muscular systems develop at a particular pace until full development is achieved by adulthood. Modern medical science has clearly identified different aspects of development that occurs from infancy to adulthood.

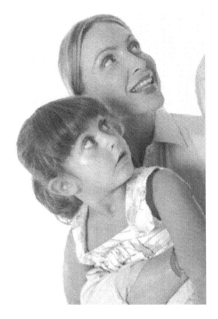

Physical development in children until adulthood

The process by which the embryo develops into a fully formed fetus and the continuation of development after birth until adulthood is reached is incredibly complex. While it is not possible to discuss the entire process in detail, here are some basic facts to understand the growth process:

The skeleton begins to form at the end of fourth week of intrauterine life.

Bones are formed by the interaction of two types of bone cells and the process continues throughout life. Collagen fibers and calcium salts are deposited around osteoblasts to form the bones. Then, osteoclasts are released from the bone marrow. They cut away the excess deposits and give shape to the bone.

At the time of birth, the formation of the skeletal system is not yet complete. The bones of the skull are not yet fused together to form the sutures. In fact, the suture between the parietal and the frontal bone of the skull closes after two years of age. The jaw structure will undergo several changes including the eruption of teeth before the adult structure is achieved. The spinal column has only two curves instead of four curves of the adult. The carpal bones are very small and do not develop before two years of age.

As the child grows, a change is clearly noticeable in the body proportions. Between age five and maturity, the basic metabolic rate falls rapidly with distinct change in the ratio between body mass and surface area.

With age, a child exhibits two types of development:

Normative development refer to those tasks that a child is normally expected to perform at a given age. It is largely dependent on culture and determines what the child can and cannot do.

The other type is the dynamic development where sequential changes occur in every aspect of functioning of the child.

Normative development is measured by growth milestone. If the baby is achieving these milestones at the appropriate time, then his growth is normal.

There is some specific pattern of development which is observed as a child grows into an adult. The large muscles of arms and legs develop first, followed by the small muscles of fingers and eyes. So, children first learn gross motor skills like running and walking. Then only do they master fine motor skills like coloring or scribbling.

Another pattern is that muscles first develop in the head region and then proceeds towards the toes. So, a child can hold up his head long before he learns to walk.

Muscles first develop in the central area and then at the edges.

Every muscle develops with the ability to perform certain general tasks. They acquire special abilities as the child grows older.

Play is an important method as well as indication of development.

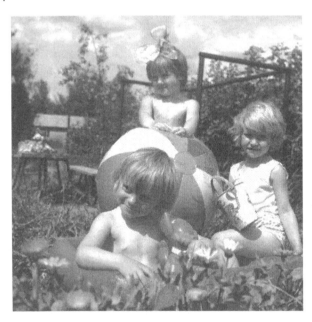

Pellegrini and Smith (1998) identified three distinct phases of activities which are vital in developing social, cognitive as well as physical skills in infants and children. These are:

Rhythmic stereotype refer to activities in infants by which they try to master the gross motor skills. Preschool age children develop strength and endurance through exercise play. This increases muscle fiber and prepares them to develop fine motor skills later. Rough and tumble play is observed in late childhood. It develops the body and also establishes boundaries of social dominance.

Growth in children occurs in spurts. Mostly, there are two spurts of rapid growth separated by two periods of slow growth. Certain skills and developments occur at certain periods of growth only.

The first spurt of rapid growth occurs from birth to about six months of age. Motor skills and muscle control develops. As the child moves from the prone to the upright position, the proportion of the body changes to accommodate the difference in posture. The skull becomes smaller in size in proportion to the body which is like the scenario in an adult. The limbs develop as the child learns to stand. Lower limbs constitute 15% of total body weight in infants but 30% in adults. This change occurs to allow the legs to carry the body weight. The center of gravity shifts downwards.

The second spurt of rapid growth is observed during adolescence. The palms and feet grow first followed by arms, legs, hip and chest. The body acquires its final shape.

The type and pace of development has definite psychological implications. For example, a school going child who can master a motor skill before his peers gets to enjoy social respect.

Similarly, children who are good at play like running, biking or climbing often attain leadership status. Thus, the neuromusculoskeletal development not only affects the physical but also the psychological aspects of the welfare of the child.

Some medical issues related to growth and development in children

Pediatric medicine emphasizes certain medical issues which are commonly observed in children and can have a long term impact on growth and development. These issues show wide variation depending on a number of factors. Racial heritage and culture definitely plays a part. Maternal health during gestation, the quality of intrauterine life, lifestyle, diet and medications are other important factors that influence these issues. The result is often some abnormality in growth or delay.

While it is not possible to list all the developmental issues that an infant or a child may have, a few are discussed here. Not only are these commonly seen, but they are intimately linked with the modern lifestyle.

Musculoskeletal pain

This is a term encompassing a wide variety of conditions. There are many reasons for chronic musculoskeletal pain among children. Some reasons are benign, being a normal part of growing up. On the other hand, in a few cases there may be a darker significance indicative of serious medical conditions. For this reason, thorough evaluation of the condition is necessary.

Parents should keep a close watch on any pain that the children may report. General observation, complete blood count, ESR, rheumatoid factor, x rays, MRI, CT scan and echocardiography are used under different circumstances to determine the actual implication of the pain. A chiropractic physician uses all these tools to make a diagnosis.

Pain which is lessened by rest coupled with absence of any abnormality in growth patterns and strength is generally benign in nature. However, if the pain is relieved by activity, aggravated by rest, there is weakness and the growth pattern is abnormal then the condition is probably more serious. The clinical examinations described above furnish the final conclusive proof in this matter.

There may be many conditions causing serious muscular pain in growing children. Possibilities of arthritis and cancer should not be ignored. Instead, laboratory tests are warranted to rule them out. One in every 6400 children are affected by cancer. Lymphoblastic leukemia is seen in one to five cases in 100000 children. Malignant tumors are another possibility.

Scoliosis

The spine of human beings is curved in a particular way so as to hold the body up against gravity. A condition which results in the abnormal curvature of the spine is known as scoliosis.

Scoliosis can develop any time before full growth is achieved. It is known as infantile scoliosis if it occurs in children up to age 3. Between ages 4 and ten, it is called juvenile scoliosis. Finally, the scoliosis that is observed between ages ten and eighteen is called adolescent scoliosis.

This condition may be congenital. Alternatively, it may be precipitated by a medical condition that creates pressure on the spine. Such conditions include cerebral palsy, polio or muscular dystrophy.

The body develops unevenly, so: shoulders may not be level; one side of the hip may be higher than another; the spine may curve more towards one side. This poor posture may lead to tiredness and pain. This may be coupled with breathing problems in some cases. The issues of confidence and social exposure gain significant importance.

If the cause is not congenital, back braces are prescribed for children above ten years of age. Surgery may be opted for in extreme conditions.

However, the above treatments are painful, time consuming and not always successful.

Juvenile rheumatoid arthritis

This is a type of autoimmune disorder that may develop as early as six months of age, but definitely before sixteen years of age.

It is a chronic condition leading to swelling and pain in the joints. The motion of that limb may become limited and the child probably stops using it to try to avoid the pain.

It can also lead to eye problems, fever, rashes and general sickliness of the constitution.

NSAIDs such as Advil are commonly prescribed accompanied by cortisone injection in extreme cases. Sometimes, disease-modifying antirheumatic drugs (DMARDs) are prescribed.

The safety as well as the efficacy of the above regime of treatment has long been questioned. Recently, several studies have been conducted showing that these traditional methods of managing this disease are yielding little result. That is why more and more people are opting for chiropractic care. Over the years, chiropractic has been seen to provide the best support and treatment for these types of ailments.

Since children are active and are learning and experimenting with a vast range of activities during their years of growth, they often injure themselves. But these activities are necessary for the proper development of the body's physiology. They are also an important means of establishing social dominance and social order. So, they cannot be restricted.

Records say that one in every three to four children are affected by trauma every year, the total number being over 22 million. The more serious ones lead to morbidity and even death.

Every year, about 2 million children aged between five and fourteen are treated for sports related injuries in America. The sports where the largest numbers of injuries are reported are basketball, cycling, soccer, and trampoline and playground activities.

In serious cases, head injuries or cardiac events are seen. Heat stroke is also another possibility. Falls and fractures are common.

It is estimated that $7.2 billion is spent each year on unintentional pediatric injuries.

Wesson and associates carried out a study which showed that 71% of seriously injured children and 54% of lightly injured children carried some physical impairment even a year after the event. The study also noted a fall in academic performance and a rise in behavioral disturbances associated with major injuries.

Prevention is better than a cure and every care should be taken to protect against the injury. Still, it is not always possible to avoid them. When they occur, it is best to consult a chiropractic physician. He uses advanced methods of general medicine, X ray and MRI to assess the damage and then uses the various methods of this discipline to stimulate the healing power of the body. This will help the child to recover in the shortest possible time.

Impact of modern lifestyle on the health of children

Lifestyles have undergone rapid and drastic changes within the past few decades. These changes are clearly visible in different areas of life. On the one hand, science and technology has made unprecedented advancements. New inventions in every sphere of life including medicine, engineering and technology have completely revolutionized the way we live. On the other hand, these huge advances in technology have not come without costs. The environment has borne most of this cost. Pollution, deforestation and other threats have increased to dangerous levels. More and more species are becoming extinct and the world stands in anticipation of disaster – whether it comes from the depletion of the ozone gas or from a nuclear or biological holocaust. The result is a strange situation in society. People are adopting a more and more consumerist lifestyle while under the constant threat of extinction!

Such social tension is bound to affect the physical and psychological health of children. Several health issues have gained predominance in recent decades which were unthinkable before. While infants have greater access to better drugs and care, children are facing unique challenges which were also not imaginable a few decades ago. It is in fact an elevated risk condition. Some of the medical issues which have become prominent in the prevailing lifestyle are as follows:

Obesity

The term obesity refers to unnatural gain in weight. This is currently one of the most serious problems threatening the children of America. Recent studies show that the problem has even begun to spread to developing countries.

In the last quarter century, the prevalence of childhood obesity has increased four times. In one study conducted in 2000, Ogden et al found that 30% of children and adolescents in America are either overweight or in danger of becoming so.

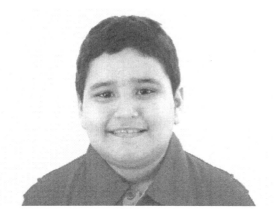

The reasons behind this trend are probably a number of psychosocial factors. On the one hand, there is probably a strong element of lack of parental attention. In the modern economy, an upwardly mobile typical American family has to rely on the income of both the partners. Rising unemployment has made the job market quite vicious. The result is that children end up being alone many times. As they have to fend for themselves, the trend of eating junk food increases more and more. Many times, the parent is also eating the same food because there is just not enough time to arrange for an alternative.

Added to this, the modern styles of games have changed considerably. Physical activities like jumping, climbing or others have largely been replaced by sedentary games concentrating on video games and computers. This has contributed towards the problem of obesity.

Childhood obesity is generally an indicator of adult obesity. It also creates a great deal of structural stress in the body. Several studies by Gushue (2005), Henderson (1992), Golan (1998) and described the different problems that may arise later in life due to childhood obesity. There is clear increase in adult osteoporosis if the person had been obese as a child.

In a study conducted in Netherlands over 2459 children between ages 2 and 17, it was found that children below 11 years of age who were obese were 1.86 times more likely to report musculoskeletal problems later in life as compared to their peers with normal weight.

Psychological issues

Pressures of modern lifestyle, neglect on the part of the parents or the primary caregiver and the highly competitive lifestyle have given rise to several psychological issues in the children of America.

As traditional patterns of games change, the feeling of isolation is intensified. Team sports like soccer or basketball have become highly competitive. Children who cannot enter this brotherhood end up feeling shaky and alone. Instead, they turn to a host of online games where make belief characters take the place of peers.

A variety of factors interact together to create a number of psychological issues in the children of today, some of which were never known before.

Immunization issues

It seems strange that any measure which is taken to protect the child from potentially life threatening condition can become an issue of contention. Yet, this is definitely the case.

On the one hand, most parents have never seen cases of the particular disease against which the child has to be inoculated. This threat never existed for their generation and they are not aware of the damage it can do. So, they are not willing to bear what they perceive as unnecessary expense.

Since 1980s, there has been an increasing trend suggesting that immunization is not only unnecessary but also potentially harmful for your child. At present, about 4500 families are suing the government because they believe a the vaccine caused harm to their children[36].

A study conducted over 10000 children found that teenagers who had received vaccines in childhood are twice more likely to suffer from autism and asthma[37] and four times more likely to suffer from attention deficit hyperactivity disorder.

Such and many other issues are the new challenges which have emerged and are facing the medical establishment today.

Role of modern medicine in dealing with the emerging issues in child health

The issues of child health, growth and development which have been emerging in the recent years have been discussed. The question remains, what is the stand of the medical establishment on these issues? How has traditional medicine responded to these emerging challenges? The following points will bring that out:

Modern medicine has definitely come up with new and more advanced treatments for the different types of health issues that children may face. Refined tests, indices and statistics are now being used for early detection of any physical problem a child may have. Immunization has advanced so much that some of the deadliest killers like smallpox and typhus have been completely eradicated from the face of the earth.

---

[36] Cbn News. Accessed May 18 2012.
http://www.cbn.com/cbnnews/204991.aspx
[37] NVIC Archives. Accessed May 18 2012. http://www.nvic.org/nvic-archives/newsletter/autismandvaccines.aspx

However, it remains open to doubt whether modern medicine has been able to respond in the optimum way to the changing health issues of children. For example, while no one doubts the success of vaccination programs, there has been an increasing trend for parents to voluntarily opt out. One such case was reported in the Vashon Islands in 2002. Here, 18% of the families enrolled in 1600 primary schools voluntarily opted out of vaccines. Parents are also concerned with the presence of elements like mercury which was used as a preservative in vaccines until 2004. Other common elements in vaccines like aluminum and monosodium glutamate have well documented health risks.

Another alarming trend is over-prescription. A study led by Adam Harsh of the University of Utah, Salt Lake City in 2011 showed that 10 million antibiotics, most of which are broad spectrum are over-prescribed annually for children. This includes antibiotics for ailments like bronchitis, flu and asthma where antibiotics actually have no role to play. The result is dangerous drug resistance which is sure to manifest later in life.

Similarly, in a study published by the Archives of General Psychiatry in 2006, it was shown that prescription of anti-psychotic drugs has increased six times between 1993 and 2002 with amphetamines increasing 120 times in the UK between 1994 and 2009. This shows that there has been a definite increase in psychiatric problems among children. However, there is also serious concern with over-prescription of these drugs which have serious side effects, affecting the heart, brain and the immune system of children.

Instances like the above are not few in number. The fact remains that modern medicine is finding it very difficult to treat all the concerns of the modern child. New techniques of medical intervention and new drugs have certainly appeared on the scene. At the same time, a huge gap has emerged in traditional medicine which has not been able to respond properly to the changing times.

Chiropractic care and child health

Traditional medicine has often failed to respond in a timely and effective way to the various ailments which children experience. That is why more and more parents are trying alternative approaches, especially chiropractic care.

In view of the over-prescription of drugs by traditional medical practitioners, chiropractic treatments have gained wide popularity. It is gentle and non invasive and mobilize the body's own strengths to deal with the various issues. Chiropractic today has come a long way from its inception in 1896. Chiropractic physicians use a variety of diagnostic tools ranging from X rays and MRI to muscle testing and kinesiology to find out whether structural misalignment or emotional complexes or chemical intrusions including allergies and nutritional deficiencies are at the root of the problem.

One of the most popular chiropractic principles believes that spinal misalignment is a major cause of many medical problems. Adjusting the spine so that it can mobilize the immunity system will be helpful in correcting any medical condition that is occurring in the body. The immune system in fact is closely related to the neural pathways. If the nervous system is disturbed because the spine is not aligned properly, this will lead to poor immune response. In his research, Ronald Pero, chief of cancer prevention researcher at New York's Preventive Medicine Institute and professor in Environmental Health at New York University concluded that chiropractic care markedly boosts the natural immune system of the body so that it can effectively fight against a number of conditions[38].

This central fact is the key to why more and more parents are opting for chiropractic care for the ailments of their children ranging from ear infection and bed wetting to ADHD and colic.

The nervous system not only dictates the immune system, it also has considerable impact on growth and development in children. So, chiropractic care is likely to provide relief to the developmental issues that children of today face.

The utility of chiropractic care lies in its various techniques which put equal emphasis on the emotional complexes created by the pressures of modern society as well as chemical elements. Methods such as neuro-emotional technique are very useful in this regard. It helps to counteract the stress caused by negative memories that are often stored in the sympathetic nervous system. They may be more harmful in children as they just may not be aware of the existence such stresses which may be the root cause of their ill health.

It is because chiropractic physicians offer holistic cure, treating not only the affected body part but also the entire physiological system that they have been found to be the most effective in the treatment of children.

[38] Fight Dr. Accessed May 18, 2012.
http://fightdr.com/information/allergens-allergies-2/

Chapter 7:

Menopause and Andropause

Menopause is often the not-talked-about stage in a women's life. It happens to most women at some point. It should not be viewed in any negative manner. Just like moving into puberty, things are changing and your course of life is going to be significantly different. However, that does not mean your health will suffer. Many women do suffer from symptoms and complications that can seem very limiting to their life quality. Men can go through a similar change in their health during this end of middle life stage. That change is called andropause. It can have many of the same or similar symptoms that women face and it seems to be even more taboo to talk about than menopause.

Both of these conditions are a natural progression of the health of an individual. Though they are different and are not something you can stop from happening, you do not have to suffer through them. As you will see, once you learn what they are, why they are happening and how to live a healthy lifestyle, your quality of life will improve vastly. The use of alternative medicine in the treatment of this condition, including the use of chiropractic care, can be the lifeline that many men and women need to get through this stage of life without feeling limited.

What Is Menopause and Why Does It Happen?

According to the National Institutes of Health, "Menopause is time in a women's life when her periods (menstruation) eventually stop and the body goes through changes that no longer allow her to get pregnant. It is a natural event that normally occurs in women age 45 to 55."[39] That seems like a simple enough definition but what it really is and how it affects a woman's life are vastly different.

When this stage of life starts, the ovaries stop producing eggs. They also stop producing the same amount of some hormones including estrogen and progesterone. The change in hormone productions is what often leads to menopausal ymptoms. The slowing of this production of hormones is due to the body no longer pushing the ovaries to produce eggs and go through the menstruation cycle. However, the process of adjustment to the lack of these hormones is often one that leads to complex symptoms in a person's life.

What Is Andropause?

Andropause is a term used to describe the onset of man-opause or male menopause. It is a menopause like condition that occurs in men as they get older. The main cause of this condition is the reduction of the production of some hormones, including testosterone. This leads to changes in a person's body and, in some men, it can lead to a new overall feeling. However, men can still reproduce during this time and afterwards. This process is not related to a shutdown of the reproductive

---

[39] PubMed health. Accessed May 11, 2012.
http://www.ncbi.nlm.nih.gov/pubmedhealth/PMH0001896/.

system. Rather, the slowing of production of these hormones is a stage of life when men begin to show signs of aging.

Because it is quite like the changes happening in women, both do have some overlap in terms of the structural and chemical changes that occur during this time. Of course, each person is a bit different.

The Changes in the Body

To fully understand what happens and what it can lead to, consider the physiological, structural and chemical changes that occur in women during menopause. Keep in mind this is a process that takes a few years to go through. It generally happens slowly.

Symptoms of Menopause

The Mayo Clinic[40] provides the symptoms of menopause to be the following:

- Irregular periods, usually slowing down in frequency
- Decreased fertility
- Vaginal dryness
- Sleep problems, in some insomnia in others a feeling of fatigue
- Hot flashes, sensations of feeling very hot very quickly
- Mood swings
- Increased abdominal fatty tissue
- Loss of the fullness of breast tissue

---

[40]Mayo Clinic. Accessed May 11, 2012.
http://www.mayoclinic.com/health/menopause/ds00119/dsection=sy mptoms.

- Thinning hair

Individuals who experience these types of changes are likely going through menopause. However, these do not often happen instantly but rather over a period of time. This often makes it harder to notice.

Symptoms of Andropause

Men also go through changes and this is often evident in the way they feel. The following are some of the most common symptoms of this change in their lives.

- Some men suffer erectile dysfunction.
- Many will have night sweats or hot flashes, though often not as significant as those women tend to have.
- Weight gain is common. The development of male breasts is also likely.
- A low libido or sex drive can occur.
- Depression and other mental health conditions occur even when not present previously.
- Some men develop hair loss.
- Sleep apnea may occur.
- Sleep related changes could occur including fatigue or irritability.

In both of these situations, menopause and andropause, the shifts are related to the hormone changes occurring in the body. Though many of these symptoms happen over time, they can still be very significant and hard to deal with for most men and women.

Managing Health

In order for the body to maintain overall health, it must balance three important components - the structural element of the body (including the actual physical aspects of the body), the chemical aspects of the body (the hormones, nutrients and even the electrical components) and the emotional/mental aspects of the body (anxiety, stress and mental health).

If you wish to overcome the symptoms of menopause or andropause, it will be necessary to improve the management of these systems. Each one has the exact level of importance the others do. If there is any weakness in one area, it directly affects the other areas. Being healthy requires the body to heal itself naturally by balancing these three components. With menopause and andropause, managing health means managing the implications of these changes on your body.

The Chemicals in the Body

The chemicals of the body change and because of this change, the body's organs and virtually every system are affected. Take a close look at why these changes occur.

The decline of reproductive hormones in women will occur beginning in the late 30's or 40's. The ovaries stop producing as much estrogen and progesterone as before because there is less of a need to regulate the menstruation cycle. These chemicals, though natural, still contribute to the overall function of the body. In simplistic terms, these hormones, which the brain directs to release, are not released because the goal is to stop being fertile.

With the reduction in these chemicals, many of the body's functions, once regulated or otherwise affected by those hormones, change. Many of the symptoms you will have are a direct result of this reduction of hormones and, at some level, the body has to get used to the new hormones present. This means that things will feel strange and your body may react negatively.

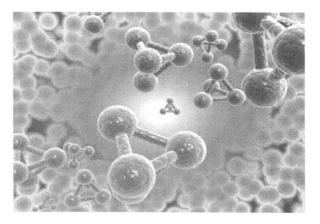

The same occurs in men with andropause. Often times, a high level of stress or other outside factors contribute to the changes and imbalances of hormones within the body. This leads to complications like those listed above. When chemicals, including these hormones, change in the body it reacts with those types of symptoms.

Chemical imbalances are the main problem. Menopause - the moving from a time when reproduction can happen to a time when it cannot - for women, should be a smooth ride. When it is not, imbalances in chemicals are leading the problem.

Getting In Balance

The goal of any treatment should be to help you to balance your hormones. As will be mentioned in just a moment, the goal of any treatment is to get you to feel normal again and to stop these symptoms. However, the right methods are important. The chemicals within the body do need regulation and balancing, but the body can do this naturally.

The Structural Impact of Menopause

As you go through menopause, your body changes and as it does, the body's structure can be negatively impacted. Though the main change is related to the chemical balances in the body, there is more to this. In short, the structure of the body can change as well. These changes often require attention and treatment to ensure you remain healthy long term.

What changes can happen? Aside from those mentioned earlier as symptoms, they may include the following:

- An increased rate of heart disease.
- Both men and women are at a higher risk of developing age-related health problems.
- Women, as well as some men, are at an increased risk of osteoporosis.
- Your body's muscles become less strong and limber. The changes can lead to a feeling of being weaker than you were.
- Some men and women begin to suffer a breakdown of systems including hearing, taste, eye sight and sex drive.

It is also possible for some health conditions to develop that could be more serious than not. Some women develop problems with fibroids. Some suffer from pelvic floor weakening. Others are at a heightened risk to develop urinary tract infections.

There are many reasons these things can develop, including the risk factor of hormonal (chemical) imbalances that protect against them. In addition, unhealthy lifestyles can also contribute.

Emotional and Mental Aspects of Menopause and Andropause

There is no doubt that the body is changing, but these changes also affect the mental health of an individual. The body is able to manage many of these ups and downs when your chemical and structural health components are maintained. However, the changes that occur during menopause can cause a variety of emotional and mental health aspects to emerge. The Cleveland Clinic[41] reports the following changes to mental health are common for men and women going through these changes:

- You may have a negative outlook on life - is this the beginning of the end? Did I want more children?

- Increased stress occurs.

- Many people suffer from depression before menopause and this worsens afterwards.

[41] Cleveland Clinic. Accessed May 11, 2012. http://www.clevelandclinic.org/health/health-info/docs/2900/2998.asp?index=10089.

- Mental health concerns can affect anyone, including anxiety.

- Your job may be changing. Your life is changing. You are apprehensive about what these changes may bring to you.

- You may have a lack of motivation even for the things you like to do.

- You may have problems concentrating.

- Mood changes are common.

- Some men become more aggressive during this period of change within their lives.

These changes, feelings and mental health changes occur because of the declining level of estrogen in the body. Menopause brings this on. For many men and women, the changes can be very limiting to their overall health. If you do face depression and anxiety, for example, this will affect your ability to be physical active. The first step is to recognize that there are changes happening within your brain that are causing these emotional changes to occur. Realize that even as much as you think they are not related to your health, they are. This is good news because it is possible to heal and overcome these limitations and get back to living the type of life you want to live. It is not possible to go back into a state of reproduction, but that is not the problem for most people. Rather, the mental and emotional health of an individual is due to the changes in the hormones in your body. Therefore, the right treatment option is often to find a way to become whole again mentally.

Traditional Medicine Approach to Treatment

Traditional medicine has a scope of options to help individuals to get through the limitations and feelings caused by menopause and andropause. There is no treatment to stop menopause from occurring. Your body will go through this process and it simply should impact you by not allowing you to reproduce any longer. However, the side effects and symptoms shift your outlook on life and cause physical manifestations. You do not need to suffer through these transformations in your body. The right treatment can help you to avoid the onset of further complications.

In healthy people, the symptoms of menopause do not last and most women are only mildly affected by them. Even in andropause, many men have minimal experiences with severe symptoms. In people who are otherwise healthy - with a balance of structural, chemical and emotional health - the body does not really need any help in getting over the symptoms or problems. It does this on its own and without any requirement for you to seek out significant treatment.

For others, however, the symptoms are significant and that means treatment is necessary. You can seek out the help of a traditional doctor to help you get back on track if you desire to do so. However, medical doctors can only provide so much help. Often, these doctors focus on the goal of treating the symptoms (rather than the underlying problem.)

Menopausal Hormone Therapy, MHT

The Office of Women's Health[42] reports that menopausal hormone therapy, or MHT, is one of the most common forms of treatment for women who are experiencing menopausal symptoms that are severe. This is a type of hormone therapy. Individuals take estrogen and progesterone - the hormones the body stops producing naturally during menopause. It promises to help with relief from many of the symptoms of moderate to severe menopause. It can also be helpful in reducing or preventing bone loss.

This treatment option does have risks including the risk of heart attacks, blood clots, strokes and breast cancer. It can help by reducing night sweats, hot flashes and sleep problems. It can help to stop vaginal dryness and discomfort. It may also help improve mood swings or depressive conditions.

There are various studies that seem to indicate that this type of treatment is not effective and imposes significant risks to the health of women. The Kronos Early Estrogen Prevention Study[43], for example, notes that there is a significant risk to a women's heart after she takes estrogen and progesterone supplements and replacements.

The Journal of the American Medical Association[44] also notes there is a higher risk of stroke, endometrial cancer, hip fracture,

---

[42] Womens Health. Accessed May 11, 2012.
http://www.womenshealth.gov/publications/our-publications/fact-sheet/menopause-treatment.cfm#h .
[43] Informa Healthcare. Accessed May 11, 2012.
http://informahealthcare.com/doi/abs/10.1080/13697130500042417.
[44] Resnick, Susan A., and Victor W. Henderson. JAMA. Accessed May 11, 2012. http://jama.ama-assn.org/content/288/17/2170.short.

pulmonary embolism, coronary heart disease, invasive breast cancer and even death as a result of taking hormone replacement therapies.

In short, this treatment option poses a significant amount of risk. It does not work for all women.

Other Treatment Options

There are other treatment options that medical doctors can offer to women who are struggling with moderate to severe symptoms from menopause. Some of these may also work for andropause suffers. However, these treatments only treat the symptoms of the condition and many also have severe side effects:

- The use of low dose antidepressants is one option. The use of antidepressants such as Venlafaxine is used. These selective serotonin reuptake inhibitors or SSRIs, have had some success in reducing hot flashes. In one study, conducted by the Archives of Internal Medicine, women who take antidepressants for post-menopausal symptoms have a 32 percent higher risk of death from all causes and a 45 percent increase in strokes than those that do not.[45]

- The use of a drug called Gabapentin is another option. Also known as neurontin, this drug is used to treat seizures. It can help to reduce hot flashes. The FDA

---

[45] The Guardian. Accessed May 11, 2012.
http://www.guardian.co.uk/lifeandstyle/2009/dec/14/menopause-pills-stroke-risk-study.

warns that those taking this medication have a higher risk for having suicidal thoughts.

- Clonidine or catapres is a type of medication given in pill or patch form. It is usually used to treat high blood pressure in medical applications. However, it can significantly reduce hot flashes. The side effects of this drug are common and include weakness, dry mouth, constipation, nervousness, decreased sexual ability and others, reports the US National Library of Medicine[46].

- Bisphosphonates are a non-hormonal medication. Some of these include Fosamax, Actonel and Boniva. These are meant to treat osteoporosis, which can increase in risk after menopause especially in women. This has become the main treatment for osteoporosis in many women and men. There are side effects including hypocalcaemia, skin rashes, inflammation and others.

What is important to know about any of these treatment options is that the goal is to reduce hot flashes or to reduce the instances of osteoporosis. However, these treatment options only treat the actual symptoms. They do not stop what is causing the hot flashes from being a problem. They just turn off the body's response to those problems (the hot flashes). For individuals who wish to truly improve their overall health, there are options to consider.

---

[46] Medline Plus. Accessed May 11, 2012.
http://www.nlm.nih.gov/medlineplus/druginfo/meds/a682243.html#side-effects.

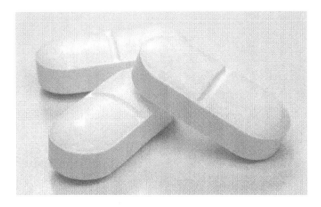

Medical science focuses only on treating these symptoms. Turn the symptoms off and the person is back to normal. That's not really how it works and, as you can see from the above, most of these treatments come with some very significant risk factors. It is a lot to take in for most people.

Individuals who want to overcome the symptoms and physical, emotional and chemical problems associated with menopause and andropause need to seek out a better solution. There are options including alternative treatments that can have a significant impact on your overall health and well being.

For example, chiropractors can recognize, diagnose, correct and support adrenal insufficiency in men and women. This is the most common cause of menopause and andropause symptoms. In addition, chiropractic physicians use various techniques to help balance hormones naturally - without the use of harmful medications or other solutions that fail to work without side effects.

Chiropractic and Alternative Medicine Care

Instead of focusing on overcoming symptoms, chiropractic care and alternative medicine focuses on solving the problem. It is not possible to stop menopause itself, but it is very possible to improve the balance of health in the body with the goal of reducing the problem. By addressing the problems associated with the body's health limitations it is possible to get back to living a healthy life.

Dealing with the cause of the problem is not as difficult as you may imagine. That is because the body has a powerful ability to heal itself. It is not possible, however, for individuals to force this to happen with the use of chemical based medicines or surgeries. Rather, you need to balance the three elements of health within the body.

As mentioned previously, to be healthy, individuals need to balance the structural, chemical and the emotional/mental health aspects. By doing this, individuals can overcome virtually any type of health concern, including the complications that arise from menopause and andropause. The question many people have, then, is how they can achieve these goals.

How Chiropractic Care Can Help

Chiropractic care can help with the improving of this balance within the body. This type of care deals specifically with the nervous system. That system is made up of a complex network of nerves that run from the brain to virtually every area of the body. These nerves serve as roads that allow messages, sent as electrical pulses and chemicals, to travel from the brain to the body's organs, muscles and other systems.

The nervous system plays an important role in regulating chemicals including hormones. In short, the nervous system, which includes the spine, will face stressful situations which can then irritate the spine and cause a decrease in the function of the nerves. When this happens, the controlling elements for the production of estrogen and progesterone are interfered with leading to the symptoms you may feel. Many stressors can cause this, such as simply sitting too long or eating the wrong foods.

With chiropractic care, you can improve the condition by finding the problem area and fixing it. One way to fix it is to use a process called an adjustment. The first step in this process is to identify the area of the body where the problem is occurring. This problem is a blockage of communications. This is called subluxation. When this blockage is present, it stops the communication from the brain from occurring. In menopausal women, this can lead to a decrease in the production of the hormones your body still needs. By using an adjustment, which is a means of manipulating the body's joints and bones, it is possible to open up that communication pathway again to allow for the brain to take over the healing process.

Subluxation removal by a chiropractor will allow for the hormonal system to begin functioning as it is supposed to work. This allows for many of the problems you feel including the moderate to severe symptoms of menopause to become improved.

Other Treatment Solutions

Subluxation treatment is one option for chiropractic physicians to use, but it is far from the only one. Your professional will want to balance those three areas. To do that, he or she must first understand what your conditions are and then offer treatment for it. Testing is often a first step. Chiropractic care, as a form of alternative medicine, has the ability to use some of the tests your medical doctor can use including EKG's, EEG's, ultrasounds, x-rays, MRI's, CAT scans and many other tests that they do not, including hair and saliva testing, to determine what the cause of the problem is. From there, the right treatment can be applied.

Treatment for menopausal symptoms may include things like the following:

- The balance of a healthy lifestyle through lifestyle coaching can help. This includes treatments that include discovery of any outside factors that are contributing to your lack of health.

- Acupuncture can also be helpful. Acupuncture, done by a professional, can work to restore the flow of blood through the body in the proper form. It is a blockage of this normal flow of blood that can lead to many of the symptoms individuals feel.

- Often times, your diet causes the chemical imbalances you feel. If your body is not getting the nutrients it needs this can lead to complications of all sorts. Nutritional supplementation can be one way that your alternative medicine treatment works for you.

The Mayo Clinic[47] reports that the use of phytoestrogens may be one of the best ways to improve menopausal symptoms. These are estrogens found in some foods naturally. Soybeans, whole grains, chickpeas and legumes have a large amount of these nutrients in them. By consuming these products, naturally or in a supplement form, you could see significant improvement in your symptoms.

Other treatments encouraged as alternative treatments by the Mayo Clinic include the use of Vitamin E to relieve mild hot flashes, black cohosh for treating hot flashes and the use of yoga to improve hot flashes and muscle changes.

In a study by the Journal of the British Menopause Society[48], the use of red clover isoflavone supplements was proven to provide a positive effect on individuals. It was show to improve bone loss, cardiovascular health and may help fight against cancer. It can also decrease the intensity and the number of hot flashes individuals have. In the study, after eight weeks of using this type of product, the participants saw a 58 percent decrease in the number of hot flashes they suffered.

What You Can Do

Individuals experiencing the symptoms of andropause or menopause do not have to suffer through these problems.

[47] Mayo Clinic. Accessed May 11, 2012.
http://www.mayoclinic.com/health/menopause/DS00119/DSECTION=alternative-medicine.
[48] Menopause International. Accessed May 11, 2012.
http://mi.rsmjournals.com/content/14/1/6.full.

Rather, they can take steps to actively improve their condition. Avoid the use of traditional medicine because of the side effects and limited function of hormone replacement therapy. Instead, turn to alternative medicine as a treatment and solution to the problem.

The difference in seeing a medical doctor and seeing a chiropractic physician is that the latter is going to solve the underlying problem contributing to the way you feel. In doing so, he or she will help your body start to heal. The healing process is very powerful and can be one of the best ways to improve your quality of life. It does not offer any side effects but it is one of the most effective solutions for overcoming menopausal complications and symptoms.

Chapter 8:

Aging

According to USA Today, Americans will spend $80 billion now and more than $114 billion by 2015 on anti-aging products.[49]

No matter if you ever pick up a wrinkle cream or have cosmetic surgery, aging is a very dominant part of life and one that starts its progression right at the start.

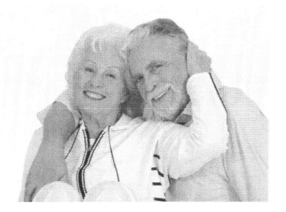

---

[49] Crary, David. "Boomers will be spending billions to counter aging." USA Today. Accessed May 10, 2012.
http://www.usatoday.com/news/health/story/health/story/2011/08/Anti-aging-industry-grows-with-boomer-demand/50087672/1.

Whether you know it or not, aging changes the physiology of your body.

Though it is possible to slow the symptoms and results of aging, it is not possible to overlook the simple fact that your body changes significantly throughout your life.

Progression of Humans - Developmental to Elderly Stages

As we are born, we begin a new life. There is no way to know what will be in that life, no idea which hardships we will have to stumble over and deal with throughout the process. However, one thing is clear. Your body begins the process of aging just as soon as you are born.

What changes? Every organ system undergoes some physiological change throughout the aging process. Consider the following examples:

- Your heart output decreases as you get older.
- Your blood pressure is on the rise as you age.
- Arteriosclerosis develops over time.
- Your lungs change and, as you get older, impaired gas-exchange occurs, in which your expiratory flow rates fall.
- Your skin even changes and loses collagen.

These are just a handful of the many transformations that do happen. But why? Why do these things have to happen? Later, we will discuss how alternative medicine helps reduce these instances to provide better function in every system.

According to The Merck Manual Home Health Handbook, "The body changes with aging because changes occur in individual cells and in whole organs. These changes result in changes in function and in appearance." Consider what this means based on the changes of cells and organs.

Aging Cells

When your cells age, they begin to function less properly than when they are new. Old cells die off and new ones replace the old cells. This is a normal part of the body's function. It happens every second in thousands of areas of your body. Why do they die?:

- In some cases, your genes tell cells when to die. A process is triggered and when that occurs, the death of the cell occurs. This is called apoptosis.
- They die because they can only divide a number of limited times. This limit is dependent on what the genes say. When cells cannot divide any longer, they get larger and then die. The mechanism that limits this is telomere.
- Damage to the cell can result in immediate death of that cell. Radiation, sunlight and even drugs can kill cells. When this happens, the function of the cell can no longer occur and, as a result, the cell dies. This is caused by free radicals.

Cells die as a normal part of life, but because they divide rapidly, there are usually plenty of new cells to do the job of the old cells.

Aging Organs

The second way in which people will age is in the organs themselves aging. The way in which an organ works is very dependent on the way in which the cells within them are working. As noted, as a cell gets older it stops functioning as well. In some organs, when cells die they are not replaced. This means that when cells in these organs die the organ's makeup changes as well:

- Ovaries
- Liver
- Kidneys
- Testes

Some of the organs do not have dividing cells. Over time, the number of cells decrease and, at some point, the level is low and that leads to the decreased function of the organ.

However, not all organs will lose a significant number of cells. The brain is one of them. As you get older, your brain is not losing a large number of cells. However, when a loss does happen, as the result of a stroke, Alzheimer's disease or Parkinson's disease the impact is substantial and lasting.

When one organ begins to stop working properly, as it is losing cells that are not replaced, this can affect other organs. For example, if the blood vessels narrow due to the development of a condition like atherosclerosis this can cause the kidneys to stop working properly over time because they are not getting enough blood flow.

Where Is This Happening?

Throughout your body, the aging process is occurring and affecting every function of your system. However, the extent of the aging process and programming of your genes are linked:

- Most organs peak at their performance shortly before you turn 30 years old.
- In most cases, the musculoskeletal system is the first area in which people notice the aging process taking hold of them.
- The eyes are often then affected.
- The ears then become affected as a person gets older.
- Internal functions will decline, as you get older, especially as you move into your elder years.

Why, is your body at 40, 50 and even 60 still looking great and functioning as it should? That is because, although the aging process and a slow decline of function is occurring, most organs of the body are built with significantly higher functional capacity than the body requires.

Why do some 30 year olds suffer from significant aging? The most common reason for loss of function in old age is not the aging process itself, in the decreasing cellular function, but rather due to various disorders.

The Consequences of Aging

Although most function of the body is maintained and remains adequate, the decline in function does have consequences. Older people:

- Are unable to handle various physical stresses as well as younger ones.
- Physical activity is reduced.
- Changes that are extreme in temperatures affect older people more so than others.
- Disorders are more common in older people.
- Older people, as a result of the aging process, are more likely to experience side effects from medications they take.

How does aging affect the functions of your body and its makeup?

Structural Changes from Aging

The structural components of the body include orthopedic, musculoskeletal, joints, muscles, spine, and bone health overall. Many changes can occur here, as discussed above.

In bones and joints, the bones tend to become less dense, weaker and even more likely to fracture. This often occurs, especially in women, due to weakness caused by a deficiency in calcium and Vitamin D. The vertebrae at the very top of the spine can cause the head to tip forward. Cartilage in the joints thins out often due to wear and tear from years of use. The ligaments of the system become less elastic and make joints feel stiffer.

Then, there's the muscular makeup. The amount of muscle tissue and its strength is reduced through aging processes. You begin to lose muscle mass around the age of 30. By 75, the amount of muscle mass your body has is about half of what it was when you were in your 20's.

Other changes include:

- The eyes change and vision weakens.
- The ears become less able to hear as well as they once did.
- The mouth and the nose are affected in that the ability to taste and smell changes and diminishes over time, especially after age 50.
- The skin becomes thinner and more elastic, usually from exposure to the sun as well as a loss of collagen production.

The body's makeup changes throughout, with each organ experiencing some level overall.

Chemical Changes from Aging

The chemical components of your body will change as you get older as well. The chemicals of your body include the foods you take in, vitamins, herbs, allergies and other components that make up the chemical composition of the body. Chemicals are a key aspect of the body's makeup in that they control the functions of virtually every organ in your body.

There are many examples of how and why this happens:

- In some people, the function of organs can contribute to the lack of proper chemical composition. For example, if your brain suffers a stroke this will affect, in some cases, the regulation of chemicals in the body, affecting other organs.
- A lack of vitamins and nutrients in the body will affect it. If older people do not get more of the nutrients they need, this will affect the function of every cell within

the body. Cells can be damaged or may not remain in their new condition as long.

- Metabolic changes in the body also occur. Those change the makeup of the system.
- The failure of the body to repair molecular damage from various processes can also play a role in how fast the body ages.

The chemical makeup of the body and the way in which those chemicals are regulated affect how the body ages.

Emotional Changes from Aging

The aging process affects the body's emotional state and the mental makeup of the system as well. How significant this is depends on various factors. It is important to note, however, that the physiological functions of aging will happen, but this does not mean that extreme disability will occur when you reach old age. In other words, mental disorders are not an inevitable part of aging, notes US Public Health Service.[50]

Aging does affect the emotional and mental health of the individual. As mentioned previously, most of the changes of the body occur from damage or disorders, including strokes and diseases. The brain, as noted, is not one of the organs that sees a significant loss of brain cells as it gets older, despite being affected by disorders.

What can happen to the brain during the aging process?:

---

[50] General Psychology. Accessed May 10, 2012.
http://webspace.ship.edu/cgboer/genpsyaging.html.

- The most common cause of change in older people is stroke. It can cause confusion, disorientation and multi-infarct dementia.
- Alzheimer's disease is another common cause of limitations. This mental disorder occurs gradually and doctors do not fully understand why it does cause severe mental limitations.
- Depression and anxiety are also a part of the aging process. This is often caused by an imbalance in the chemicals in your brain.
- Functions of the body are controlled by this as well. The libido of men and women, for example, changes. This occurs due to the changes in the chemicals produced in the brain.

It is important to note that any limitation that occurs, including the structural, chemical and emotional aspects of aging, can be improved upon by improving diet, exercise and overall health. Balancing these three factors - chemical, structural and emotional health - can reduce the effects of aging on the body and mind.

Can Humans Really Live Longer?

Considering that the body is preprogrammed through genes to cause cells to die, it may not seem like there is a way to live longer. Isn't it already preprogrammed into a person's code? There is evidence that tells scientists that it is possible to live a longer life. The reasons are numerous, in fact.

Genes Are a Part of It

Thomas Perls of the Boston University School of Medicine[51] published a study that provides information on if a person will live longer. In the study, the researchers were able to predict if a person will live to be 100 with 77 percent accuracy by just studying the genes of the body. Those who make it to a very old age do so, the study indicates, not only because of the healthy aging process but also because of their genome makeup.

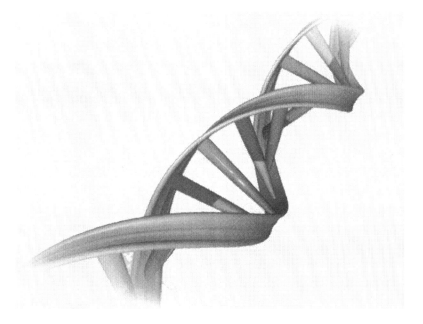

[51] Boston University School of Public Health. Accessed May 10, 2012. http://sph.bu.edu/index.php?Itemid=366&articleid=2941&id=623&option=com_insidernews&task=view.

The California Pacific Medical Center Research Institute[52] also conducted a study on this topic. It showed that human longevity is partly inheritable. How is this possible? The report indicates that the longevity genes that all people have built into them might slow the rate of age-related changes in your body's cells.

By improving the functional aspects of the cell and their programming, these genes can help increase the resistance of the cells against environmental stress factors. This includes giving the body a better ability to fight off infection and injury or reduce the onset of many types of age related conditions.

Those Genes Need Help

Individuals who want to live longer have to give their body the very functional aspects it needs in order to get healthy and to maintain health. In other words, if you do not provide your body with the balance of health in the structural, chemical and emotional aspects, even genes cannot allow you to live longer.

It is important for individuals to take an active role in creating a long life by improving their overall health. By striving for health, it may be possible to allow those longevity genes to work for you to extend your life.

Is It Possible to Age Gracefully?

There are two ways to look at the term aging gracefully. For some people, this term means that individuals should take the aging process in stride because it is a normal part of life. Instead of fighting the aging process, individuals should accept it in a

---

[52] Warren S.Browner etal. Longevity Consortium. Accessed May 10, 2012. http://www.longevityconsortium.org/resources/publications/the_genetics_of _human_longevity.pdf.

graceful manner and adapt to it. While this is a very good step to take for some people, it should not be taken to mean there is nothing you can do to slow the aging process significantly.

A second way to look at this term is to consider what the aging process does to the body and then to indicate ways to slow that progression. For example, you can age slowly and without a big impact on your overall health and well-being. Instead of aging quickly and feeling, looking or experiencing the effects of aging as a large impact, you may be able to slow down aging significantly and thus live a longer, healthier life.

Aging gracefully should be your goal. It is clear that we cannot turn off our genes and live as long as we want. However, it is possible to give your body everything it needs to minimize the effects of aging and even help those genes to keep you living a long life.

Why Is This So Hard?

Why does it seem that living a long life is so hard to do? Most people do not live in the inner city where violence is a big factor in their everyday lives. In the United States, most people have access to good quality health care that helps individuals to at least improve their diseases or illnesses. A simple fracture does not kill Americans as it might kill those in third world countries. Yet, for some reason, there is still an incredible lack of ability to live longer.

In 2011, the Huffington Post[53] published information regarding the countries with the longest life span. Unfortunately, the

---

[53] Friedman, Howard S. Huffington Post. Accessed May 10, 2012. http://www.huffingtonpost.com/howard-steven-friedman/life-expectancy_b_867361.html#s284378&title=5_Sweden_814.

United States did not make it into the list of the top five countries:

1. In Japan, the average life span is 82.7 years.
2. In Switzerland, the average life span is 82.2 years.
3. In Australia, the average life span is 81.5 years.
4. In Italy, also tied with Australia, the average life span is 81.5 years.
5. In Sweden, people live to 81.4 years on average.

Where is the United States in this ranking? It falls back considerably with the average life expectancy of about 78 years. It is comparable to that of people who live in Cuba. The US is behind Mexico, Poland, the Slovak Republic, Turkey, Hungary and the Czech Republic.

People do not want to learn about these figures, but they are very real. Aging in the United States happens because of the simple lack of health due to the lifestyles people here have.

Unhealthy Lifestyle Choices

One of the most common problems for individuals who are facing a short lifespan is the unhealthy lifestyle they are living. The following factors are some of those:

- People are obese. The Centers for Disease Control and Prevention note that 1/3 of all adults in the United States are obese. Obesity contributes to many health problems including heart disease, hypertension and diabetes.

- People do not get physical exercise. To keep the structural components of your body functioning, as they should be, you simply must utilize exercise as a daily component. Many people get no physical exercise daily.

- The use of tobacco products, illegal drugs and excessive alcohol also contribute to the underlying problem. It can be a very large part in reducing the lifespan of an individual.

These are just some of the reasons that people do not live as long as they could. Aging is hastened in these situations.

Failure of Medical Health Care

Another element that contributes to the shortened lifespan and the rapid aging of Americans is the poor medical health conditions. Though emergency room treatment is stellar, the overall treatments received by medical doctors are lacking. In short, medical doctors often treat just the symptoms of the problem without actually solving the underlying cause. This leads to a complex problem for many individuals - they feel better but really have no improvement in the cause of their ailment.

Traditional medicine uses chemical-based drugs and treatments that focus on the symptoms of a condition rather than the actual underlying problem. As a result, traditional medicine is unable to provide individuals with the health they are seeking. Traditional medicine does not focus on healing but just on treating what it can see. This is another reason why Americans age so much faster than other countries that incorporate alternative medicines as a simple, effective component of healing.

Chiropractic Care and Alternative Medicine Slows Aging

It is possible to make significant improvements in your health and to encourage the body to remain healthy. The goal is to balance the three components of health - chemical, emotional and structural health. When these three elements are balanced properly, the result is the ability to heal and be healthy (not just to cover up the symptoms of ailments).

How can this happen? The use of alternative medicine is a critical component of the process. In many ways, by treating the body with natural elements and methods will make the biggest difference. The goal of alternative medicine should be to achieve a balance of those three components. There are many ways that alternative medicine can do just that.

Chiropractic Treatment

One of the ways in which alternative medicine can be helpful is in the use of chiropractic treatment of subluxations. The goal is to restore the body's health by improving the nervous system function. Your brain is at the helm and nerves that travel down the spinal column to each of your body's organs and systems are the pathways. The problem is many people have roadblocks in these pathways.

With subluxations, this roadblock stops the body from communicating properly. With traditional chiropractic care, there is the ability to remove any limitations and to allow for the restoration of the communication of the nervous system. In other words, the brain knows when there is a problem and can address the problem right away with its natural ability to heal.

This is not possible when individuals are facing a blockage of this nervous system passageway.

Chiropractic care improves that function and, therefore, can allow the body's natural healing process to take place. Through an adjustment of the spinal column or to other areas of the body where a subluxation is occurring, chiropractors can give the body back the ability to heal. To heal, it needs to balance the three components of health.

However, chiropractic care goes farther than this. It is a combination of alternative medicines to improve aging. In the subluxation treatment option, the body's functions and its ability to fight off external problems is improved through adjustments. This means your body can look and feel younger because the cells remain healthy.

Additional Alternative Treatments for Improving Aging from Chiropractors

Other alternative treatments available from chiropractic physicians can help to improve the aging process. Remember, it is not possible to stop aging since many cells are programmed to live only a set amount of time. Organs break down over time. However, it is possible to control the effects of the world around that. This can be done by focusing on all of the alternative treatments that help to balance the three elements of health - chemical, structural and emotional.

The following are some examples of how this is done. Through professional help from chiropractic physicians, individuals can learn better what their options are. These are some solutions offered by modern chiropractors today:

- Acupuncture - This is a method used to restore the healthy flow of blood through the body. It is not painful but it can improve a person's blood flow by removing blockages. By doing this, the body's natural healing processes can work as they are meant to.
- Lifestyle Coaching - This is a very important component to being healthy today and it is one in which most people are lacking. In short, you need to know what you are doing that is negatively affecting your health so that you can remove that problem. In doing this, you allow the natural healing of the body to take place.
- Nutritional - Often times, there is a great need for supplementing as well as to improve overall health and well-being through diet. The foods people eat are lacking the nutrition that the systems of the body, including the cells, need in order to maintain function and health. By improving the nutritional components of the body, individuals will see a significant improvement in health.
- Physical - There is the necessity to improve all forms of physical health including through active and passive methods. Are you exercising? Are you filling the needs of your body's physical demands? If not, this could be an underlying problem as well.

It is possible to see significant improvement in your overall health but it is not possible to do this if you do not take on these alternative treatment options. In short, your body will age if it is not healthy. It will age far faster and sooner than it should if and when you are dealing with an unhealthy lifestyle. Traditional medicine does not do enough to improve the functions of the body or to address the underlying cause of the problem.

How Chiropractors Can Help Slow Aging

Chiropractic care addresses the causes of your rapid aging. As noted, Americans tend to live a shorter life due to their environment, lack of quality medical care and due to lifestyle choices. With the aid of a chiropractic physician, you can see significant improvement in your health.

These professionals will use numerous tests to determine what the problems may be. This includes tests related to blood work, EEGs, EKG's, diagnostic ultrasounds, hair testing, saliva testing and numerous others to determine what the problem is. Once this occurs, the professional will then use the proper forms of alternative medicine to address the underlying problem. Note that this has nothing to do with making you feel better or to make you look better right away. Rather, it has to do with solving the cause of your problems.

With proper chiropractic care, individuals will see their body restored to health. A balance is in place between the structural, emotional and chemical makeup of the body. As such, the body can naturally heal itself and overcome many of the premature aging factors affecting it.

If you want to look and feel younger and live a longer, healthier life, the only thing you can do is to restore the balance of health within your body. Using alternative medicine to do this is critical. In doing so, you will see a significant improvement in your energy levels, the way your skin looks, the way your joints move and even in your emotional health. You do not have to be a victim of premature aging.

Bibliography

NCBI. Accessed May 15, 2012.
   http://www.ncbi.nlm.nih.gov/pubmed/1548898

JStor.org. Accessed May 15, 2012.
   http://www.jstor.org/discover/10.2307/4372130?uid=37382
   56&uid=2&uid=4&sid=47698967570967

Natural Health Information Center. Accessed May 15, 2012.
   http://www.natural-health-information-centre.com/modern-
   medicine.html

SciDev. Accessed May 15, 2012.
   http://www.scidev.net/en/health/antibiotic-
   resistance/opinions/biomed-analysis-end-complacency-on-
   drug-resistance-1.html

SciDev. Accessed May 15, 2012.
   http://www.scidev.net/en/health/antibiotic-
   resistance/news/sleeping-sickness-drug-resistance-
   mechanism-identified.html

Web.Me. Accessed May 15, 2012.
   http://web.me.com/stevescrutton/Banned_Pharma_Drugs/
   Prozac-Seroxat.html

Think Quest. Accessed May 15, 2012.
   http://library.thinkquest.org/24206/chiropractic.html

Wikipedia. Accessed May 15, 2012.
   http://en.wikipedia.org/wiki/Chiropractic

Mayo Clinic. Accessed May 15, 2012.
   http://www.mayoclinic.com/health/chiropractic-
   adjustment/MY01107/DSECTION=why-its-done

Web Medical Directory. Accessed May 15, 2012.
http://www.webmd.com/heartburn-gerd/treating-acid-reflux-disease-with-diet-lifestyle-changes

Web Medical Directory. Accessed May 15, 2012.
http://www.webmd.com/heartburn-gerd/treating-acid-reflux-disease-with-diet-lifestyle-changes

Holistic Healing. Accessed May 15, 2012.http://www.holistic-mindbody-healing.com/allopathic-medicine.html

Canadian Women's Health Network. Accessed May 15, 2012.
http://www.cwhn.ca/en/node/42145

NCBI. Accessed May 15, 2012.
http://www.ncbi.nlm.nih.gov/pubmed/17327577

Scientific American. Accessed May 15, 2012.
http://www.scientificamerican.com/article.cfm?id=why-women-report-being-in

Beth Israel Deaconess Medical Center. Accessed May 15, 2012.
http://www.bidmc.org/YourHealth/HealthNotes/BonesandJoints/SportsInjuriesandPrevention/WomenandSportsInjuries.aspx

LiveStrong.com. Accessed May 15, 2012.
http://www.livestrong.com/healthy-diet-plan/

Allergic Living. Accessed May 15, 2012.
http://allergicliving.com/index.php/2010/11/20/allergies-why-so-many-now/?page=3

National Institute of Mental Health. Accessed May 15, 2012.
http://wwwapps.nimh.nih.gov/health/publications/the-numbers-count-mental-disorders-in-america.shtml

E-Medicine Health. Accessed May 15, 2012.
http://www.emedicinehealth.com/thyroid_problems/article_em.htm

New York College of Health Professions. Accessed May 15, 2012.
http://www.nycollege.edu/health-care-clinics/our-holistic-approach.php

Hormone Health Network. Accessed May 15, 2012.
http://www.hormone.org/endo101/.

Human Fertisilation & Embryology Institute. Accessed May 15, 2012.
http://www.hfea.gov.uk/fertility-treatment-risks.html.

Mercola.com. Accessed May 15, 2012.
http://articles.mercola.com/sites/articles/archive/2010/03/3
0/there-are-too-many-preventable-deaths-among-new-moms.aspx.

Schlaud, M, and W J. Kleeman. International Journal of Epidemiology.
Accessed May 15, 2012.
http://ije.oxfordjournals.org/content/25/5/959.full.pdf.

Science Daily. Accessed May 15, 2012.
http://www.sciencedaily.com/releases/2010/08/100817111
658.htm.

Child Health USA 2004. Accessed May 17, 2012.
http://www.mchb.hrsa.gov/mchirc/chusa_04/pages/0405ii
mr.htm.

Clermont College. Accessed May 17, 2012.
http://biology.clc.uc.edu/courses/bio105/endocrin.htm.

HRSA. Accessed May 17, 2012.
http://www.mchb.hrsa.gov/programs/womeninfants/prenat
al.html.

Medline Plus. Accessed May 17, 2012.
http://www.nlm.nih.gov/medlineplus/healthproblemsinpreg
nancy.html.

The Ohio State University. Accessed May 17, 2012.
http://ohioline.osu.edu/hyg-fact/5000/pdf/5573.pdf.

Center for Disease Control. Accessed May 18, 2012.
http://www.cdc.gov/breastfeeding/pdf/2011BreastfeedingR
eportCard.pdf.

Mayo Clinic. Accessed May 18, 2012.
http://www.mayoclinic.com/health/postpartum-
depression/DS00546/DSECTION=causes.

NIHCD. Accessed May 18, 2012.
http://www.nichd.nih.gov/health/topics/Breastfeeding.cfm.

Womens Health. Accessed May 18, 2012.
http://www.womenshealth.gov/breastfeeding/.

Berk, L.E. (1989) Child Development; Boston, Mass.: Allyn and Bacon

Payne, V. G., and L.D. Isaacs (1987); Human Motor Development: A
Lifespan Approach; Mountain View, Calif.: Mayfield.

Papalia, D. and Olds, S. (1992) Human Development, 5th edn, New
York: McGraw-Hill

Bee, H. (1995) The Developing Child, 7th edn, New York: HarperCollins

Sherry DD, Malleson PN. (2001); Nonrheumatic musculoskeletal pain,
and idiopathic musculoskeletal pain syndromes; In: Cassidy JT,
Petty RE, eds. Textbook of Pediatric Rheumatology. 4th ed.
Philadelphia, Pa.: Saunders

Calabro JJ, Marchesano JM. (1968); The early natural history of
juvenile rheumatoid arthritis. A 10-year follow-up study of 100
cases; Med Clin North Am.

Ogden CL, Flegal KM, Carroll MD, Johnson CL. (2002); Prevalence and
trends in overweight among US children and adolescents, 1999-
2000; JAMA

Clark H, Goyder E, Bissell P, et al (2007) How do parents' child-feeding behaviors influence child weight? Implications for childhood obesity policy J Public Health (Oxford)

Kent, Christopher (1996); Models of Vertebral Subluxation: A Review. Journal of Vertebral Subluxation Research; Vol 1:1.

Sternberg EM, Chrousos GP, Wilder RL, Gold PW (1992); The stress response and the regulation of inflammatory disease; Ann Intern Med

Cleveland Clinic. Accessed May 11, 2012.
http://www.clevelandclinic.org/health/health-info/docs/2900/2998.asp?index=10089.

Informa Healthcare. Accessed May 11, 2012.
http://informahealthcare.com/doi/abs/10.1080/13697130500042417.

Mayo Clinic. Accessed May 11, 2012.
http://www.mayoclinic.com/health/menopause/DS00119/DSECTION=alternative-medicine.

Mayo Clinic. Accessed May 11, 2012.
http://www.mayoclinic.com/health/menopause/ds00119/dsection=symptoms.

Medline Plus. Accessed May 11, 2012.
http://www.nlm.nih.gov/medlineplus/druginfo/meds/a682243.html#side-effects.

Menopause International. Accessed May 11, 2012.
http://mi.rsmjournals.com/content/14/1/6.full.

PubMed health. Accessed May 11, 2012.
http://www.ncbi.nlm.nih.gov/pubmedhealth/PMH0001896/.

Resnick, Susan A., and Victor W. Henderson. JAMA. Accessed May 11, 2012. http://jama.ama-assn.org/content/288/17/2170.short.

The Guardian. Accessed May 11, 2012.
http://www.guardian.co.uk/lifeandstyle/2009/dec/14/menopause-pills-stroke-risk-study.

Womens Health. Accessed May 11, 2012.
http://www.womenshealth.gov/publications/our-publications/fact-sheet/menopause-treatment.cfm#h .

Boston University School of Public Health. Accessed May 10, 2012.
http://sph.bu.edu/index.php?Itemid=366&articleid=2941&id=623&option=com_insidernews&task=view.

Crary, David. "Boomers will be spending billions to counter aging."
USA Today. Accessed May 10, 2012.
http://www.usatoday.com/news/health/story/health/story/2011/08/Anti-aging-industry-grows-with-boomer-demand/50087672/1.

General Psychology. Accessed May 10, 2012.
http://webspace.ship.edu/cgboer/genpsyaging.html.

Friedman, Howard S. Huffington Post. Accessed May 10, 2012.
http://www.huffingtonpost.com/howard-steven-friedman/life-expectancy_b_867361.html#s284378&title=5_Sweden_814.

Warren S.Browner etal. Longevity Consortium. Accessed May 10, 2012.
http://www.longevityconsortium.org/resources/publications/the_genetics_of_human_longevity.pdf.

Picture Credits:

The publisher would like to thank the following for their kind permission to reproduce their photographs:

Wikimedia Commons for public Domain Images used in various chapters of this book.

Also, more specifically, the various images below were reproduced with the permission of their respective creators:

Chapter 1:

Armillaria_ostoyae by W.J.Pilsak at the German language Wikipedia

Chapter2:

MRT_ACL_PCL_01 by Marios G Lykissas, George I Mataliotakis, Nikolaos Paschos, Christos Panovrakos, Alexandros E Beris and Christos D Papageorgiou

Chapter 3:

1000px-World_map_of_Female_Obesity,_2008.svg by Lokal_Profil

Chapter 4:

765px-Spondylolysis-_back_pain by Lparis22

347px-Month_9 by Miraceti

Chapter 6:

Children_playing - RIA Novosti archive, image 490715, S. Lidov, CC-BY-SA 3.0

All the remaining images in the book are from:

FreeDigitalPhotos.net

About the Author

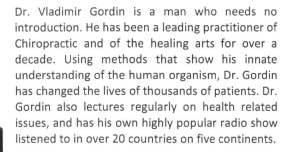

Dr. Vladimir Gordin is a man who needs no introduction. He has been a leading practitioner of Chiropractic and of the healing arts for over a decade. Using methods that show his innate understanding of the human organism, Dr. Gordin has changed the lives of thousands of patients. Dr. Gordin also lectures regularly on health related issues, and has his own highly popular radio show listened to in over 20 countries on five continents.

Dr. Gordin's qualifications include his Doctorate in Chiropractic from the prestigious National University of Health Sciences, his degrees in Biology and Physics and Human Biology, and post-graduate studies that have qualified him to be Board Eligible Diplomate in Chiropractic Orthopedics and Applied Kinesiology, as well as Board Candidate Diplomate in Clinical Nutrition. He also holds certifications that grant him mastery over a large variety of treatment protocols. His qualifications and considerable experience allow Dr. Gordin to use a vast array of highly effective methods and techniques.

*The **core** of Dr. Gordin's **philosophy** is treating the root cause of a patient's problems. His **goal** is to help his patients towards lasting and permanent health, guiding them towards a gentle, yet rapid, recovery.*

This series of books by Dr. Gordin is an expression of this philosophy and goal...

Dr. Gordin resides with his beautiful wife and three children in Chicago, IL.

Made in the USA
Las Vegas, NV
28 December 2021

39702074R00105